Crohn's Disease

CROHN'S DISEASE: The other "C" word

Crohn's Disease, Court Reporting, and Custody Battles

The Joy of Living with a Chronic Illness

Table of Contents

WHO AM I? I'm Claudia Merandi. I'm 49 years old. I'm mom to Francesca 16, and to Ava, 12.

I'm a daughter to my hero, my mom, Dottie Merandi, 82, who dedicated her life to be my caretaker, she endured endless days in the hospital, and fought a custody battle with me. She advocated for me when I couldn't. My mom is my heartbeat. There's no doubt, without my mom, I wouldn't be alive today.

I'm a blogger, author, fitness competitor, and Crohn's Warrior. My greatest passion is being an advocate for the Crohn's/Colitis community and speaking for those who have no voice.

I've had Crohn's Disease since I was a kid and developed Ulcerative Colitis four years ago. Until three years ago, I spent over 400 days in a hospital bed and endured painful surgeries, 47 CT scans, 47 MRIs, C-difficile 26 times, and too many kidney stones to count. That's the hard part of Crohn's. The easy part is the debilitating joint pain that would cripple me and fatigue which would put me in bed for days at a time.

WHY THE NAME FOR THE BOOK?

COURT REPORTING:

Court reporting played a significant part of my life. I started my business at 24 and turned it into a finely-tuned machine. I had 15 amazing reporters that I considered sisters. I was fiercely protective of my staff. They kept my secret safe for years before revealing to my clients how sick I was with Crohn's. I thrived on deadlines, chasing the lawyers to pay their bills, taking down testimony, and everything else that came along with being a reporter. We're a small community. Few people can learn a new language and take it down, on that little machine, and write 225 words per minute. We're a unique breed. I cherished my court reporters and my clients.

THE CUSTODY BATTLE.

My beautiful daughter, Francesca, was born in 2001. Her father and I had a short-lived relationship. We were very different people in every way. I take the blame for pushing a relationship that shouldn't have existed. Francesca's father is a power-driven man. He had a much grander sense of himself than the reality. He didn't believe in illness, especially mine. He would say I had a "make-believe illness," or I used the hospital for a vacation because I didn't want to deal with life.

He needed to have the power, the last word, and the ability to navigate situations in his favor. In therapy, the therapist told me he had narcissistic traits. But the most significant destruction he caused: serving me with papers for custody of my child the day I came home from the hospital with a colostomy bag. I can tell you this: when I found out I was pregnant, he warned me not to retain counsel. He vowed to make my life a living hell. I can assure you, he made good on his word.

My family unit has been destroyed because of the turmoil that came with his shenanigans. He robbed me of being a mom to my Francesca. He refused to believe when our daughter was sick and refused to accept that

I suffered from an illness. I attribute his mindset to him attending "The University of YouTube." If it was on You Tube, it had to be true.

The last time I set eyes on him was in family court. He petitioned to have our daughter taken off an acne medication she desperately needed. This was a medication prescribed by three different doctors.

When I reinvented myself, I severed ties with "custody dad" per my doctor's advice.

Fighting the custody battle and co-parenting with this man worsened my illness. To not address how the custody battle affected my illness would be erasing the 14 sickest years of my life. At times, it seemed like I was drowning. I didn't know how much I could take before I would break. I often ask myself if he is remorseful for the havoc he wreaked on my family and my relationship with our daughter. I don't believe narcissists feel remorse.

Many who follow my blog ask me if I hate this man. Absolutely not. If I hate, that means someone gets to control how I feel.

My daughter and I have a strained relationship and I wholeheartedly blame "custody dad" for that.

To my daughter, Francesca; Nana, sissy, and I love you with every fiber. I didn't write this book with malice towards your dad.

You have a positive relationship with your dad and I guess that's all that matters. I love you and I don't want you to hurt. But to be a healthy mom, I must be a happy mom. I pray that one day you and I can be whole again. You are my heartbeat.

*****

MY DAUGHTER AVA

Ava is my younger daughter. Her dad is Todd, my plumber. Todd is a good guy. He let me be a mother. He let me do my job, even from a hospital bed. Todd never once questioned a decision about Ava's wellbeing. He is a hard-working man. He never understood custody dad's antics. I prayed for years that Todd and I could reconcile, but it wasn't in God's plan. I'll always have a special place in my heart for Todd.

Ironically, both dads have the same birthday.

*****

HOW DID THE GIRLS COPE WITH A SICK MOM?

I hated that my girls had to see me in a hospital bed or be in my bed at home. I spend a lot of time in bed. But that's what this illness does. It robs you of everything. As I write this book, Ava copes with my disease differently than Francesca. I think that's because Ava's dad and I have always been on the same page. When there's something that's just a little off between two parents and a child is involved, add Crohn's into the mix, and we've got problems ahead.

When I went in the hospital, my mom cared for my girls. She is also my neighbor. My girls never missed one day of school, one doctor's appointment, or one activity when I "went in." I created my children's' lives within five minutes of my home. Their school, pediatrician, dentist, tennis, and piano lessons were within five minutes of my house. My children needed a schedule. Kids thrive with schedules. My mom played a pivotal part of their schooling and was a constant presence at their school. When they say it takes a village, they're not shitting you.

And that's where the book title originated from.

*****

IS THIS A SELF-HELP BOOK?

This is not a self-help book. However, it is how I helped myself cope with the illness that tried to rob me of my life. Some of you are reading my book because you have followed my blog, and for that, I am thankful for the support you've extended. You're all family. Hundreds of my fellow Crohnies put their trust in me and allowed me to speak for them when they had no voice. I thank you for entrusting me with some of your hardest and challenging times.

Some of you may be reading this book, on the toilet, during a flare; others may be reading it because you just found out your child was diagnosed, or some may be trying to get information to help family or friends diagnosed with the same condition.

I blogged, weekly, about Crohn's and I was also writing this book at the same time. So, for the people who don't enjoy reading long chapters, I thought, "Let's turn my blog into a book."

Ladies and gentlemen, I present to you, "Crohn's Disease, the other C WORD."

*****

Whoever you are, stay strong, stay confident as fuck, and remember… you have a friend in Providence, Rhode Island.

Now, let's get this bitch going.

A NIGHT OUT ON THE TOWN WITH CROHN'S

I'm out to dinner with my best friend, Carole Malaga. The minute I look at the menu, the rumbling begins in my stomach. I'm thinking to myself, "Oh, my God, I'm going to shit my pants." I'm just staring at the menu, trying to block out all the noise. It seems when you have a Crohn's flare, the more people talk, the worse the pain gets and you're ready to commit a heinous crime on the person sitting next to you.

I give Carole the "eye." She knows what the "eye" looks like. We go to the ladies' room and there's just one bathroom. I'm praying to God. "Oh, God, please; oh, please, don't let me shit my pants. I promise to never say the "C" word again," even though it's a favorite.

Life without the "C" word seems unimaginable. It horrifies women. I don't understand why.

Carole follows me to the bathroom to find there's only one. Who the fuck puts in one bathroom? I'm paying $26 for a bowl of pasta Bolognese, that I can't eat, and they install one bathroom. Fuckers.

I tell Carole the plan. She'll tell people that are waiting to use the bathroom that there's a plumber in there and that the bathroom is out of order.

I'm on the potty for an eternity. The pain is like labor.
Here comes the pain, then the chills, and now I'm sweating like a pig.
And then it happens: sweet Mother, Mary of Jesus, finally, relief. If this toilet doesn't flush, I'm climbing out the window. While I'm on the toilet, I'm silently taking measurements of the window to see if I can fit through it.
It flushes. Thank you, Jesus. That was a close one.
I exit the ladies room and return to the table. I'm pale, sweaty, and I decide there will be no food tonight; just a pain pill for me.
I can see the look on my mom's face. She dies just a little every time I flare. But I assure her and everyone else at the table that I'm fine. I'm always fine.
This is Crohn's Disease. People are not banging the door down to get in this club. But God enrolled me in this special club when I was six years old.

GROWING UP WITH CROHN'S

I'm eight years old and it's the most exciting time of my life. It's Saturday night. Lawrence Welk is on, followed by...wait for it...The Love Boat and Fantasy Island. My parents go out on Saturday night. I can still smell my mother's hairspray, Aqua Net.

My brother, Billy, is 18 months older than I. We had our Saturday night ritual; walk up the street to the corner store, Douglas Drug, and buy as many bags of little potato chips we could afford; Sour Cream and Onion, Barbeque, Doritos, Cheetos, and Fritos. We don't discriminate against any chip.

When we get back home, we open all the bags and empty them into a big, brown paper bag. I can still see all the grease stains on the bag. Then we shake the bag and we settle in for a night of TV.

Halfway through The Love Boat, my stomach hurts. I try and wiggle around, trying to ignore the pain. Although I'm eight-years-old, I'm already too familiar with stomach aches. I run to the bathroom and panic sets in. The pain is bad. I cry out to my brother, "Billy, get mommy." There are no cell phones in 1976.

I'm sitting on the toilet and I have a towel pressed up against my stomach. My dad told taught me that trick because he had a lot of stomach issues himself. He said it would help with the stomach pain. I remember I would get the chills, the sweats, the pain, and then relief. The relief is massive diarrhea.

I run back out and resume watching Doc and Julie McCoy.

Eating and running to the bathroom was a common occurrence from an early age.

As a kid, after dinner, I would lay my head on my dad's lap. My dad was a RIPTA bus driver. When he came home, we always sat down together for dinner. My mom cooked every night.

Ten minutes after I would eat, I would run to the bathroom. My siblings would accuse me of not wanting to do the dishes. When I was in the bathroom, I could hear my sisters say, "She just doesn't want to do the dishes."

On Sundays, my mom would make an amazing sauce filled with big meatballs, sausage, and a stick of pepperoni. And then, for the main meal, she would make a big pork roast, macaroni, and a salad. This would come to be known as the "near-death experience" meal.

On Sundays, my dad would get to the bathroom before me. He could run faster.

I remember one night sitting in the living room and seeing his bus pull up. He was running into the house. He screamed, "Claude, watch the bus. Jesus Christ, I'm going to shit my pants." Meanwhile, there was a bus full of people in front of my house. That was a good day for my dad because he made it to the bathroom. Some days the poor guy would have to go on the bus after all the passengers were off.

My dad didn't do well with the pain associated with Crohn's or Colitis. I can remember him crying in the bathroom. I would put the pillow over my ears tightly, so I couldn't hear him cry. My dad felt a tremendous sense of guilt because he assumed I inherited Crohn's from him. Crohn's, unfortunately, is very hereditary.

I never blamed my dad for my illness.

BEING A TWEEN WITH CROHN'S

When I was around 11, my mom would try and bribe me to go to the doctor's because she knew something was wrong. She had my grandmother (her mother) show me her bag. (WARNING: THIS WON'T ENTICE YOUR KID TO GO SEE A GI DOC).

I didn't like going to my grandmother's house. If I was in the bathroom, I could hear my Nana say, "Babe, something's wrong with this kid. She's always in the bathroom."

My mom was an identical twin and each twin was called Babe. They looked so much alike, I couldn't tell them apart without my glasses. I was nearsighted and had thick glasses. I was fortunate, enough, to inherit that trait, along with Crohn's, from my dad. But the two best traits that I inherited from my dad were cystic acne and my sense of humor.

By the time I was 12, I assumed every kid had gone to the bathroom twenty times a day and had diarrhea. When a doctor would ask, "Claudia, didn't you think it's unusual to have diarrhea," I would reply, "How would I know?"

At 12, I had my first sigmoidoscopy. I was crying for my mom when the prick doctor was doing the scope. There was no sedation. My mother almost broke the door down. The doctor diagnosed me as having a "nervous stomach."

Eventually, barium enemas, scopes, CT scans, all became the norm. My dad would try and bribe me with McDonald's if I could just get through one barium enema without jumping off the table. I never succeeded. A trip to McDonald's wasn't worth it.

As a teen, I never thought of myself as sick. Crohn's or Colitis was not even mentioned. Nobody knew about the mysterious illness that would plague my dad and me. I think I just blocked out all the years of pain and running to the bathroom because I never thought of myself as sick.

THE BEGINNING OF MY CROHN'S CAREER AND STRESS

After graduating from high school, I went to work on cruise ships. My Crohn's flares were still under control during this time. I was still eating whatever I wanted and running to the bathroom immediately after. I came out of remission only one time during this period.

Eventually, I decided on a career as a court reporter. People would mention how nobody ever graduated and that I would be stuck in school forever.

Once I started school, I fell in love with it. I was up for the challenge. Becoming a reporter is like learning a foreign language and learning to "take" testimony down on that little machine you see in the courtroom. We had to retain up to five minutes' worth of testimony.

The stress involved with becoming a reporter was off the charts. Some girls would be in school for four or five years. It's a tough gig.

I got ill when I was ready to complete my degree. This would become the first violent attack, leaving me traumatized.

The pain was so severe that I couldn't stop vomiting. If I looked at food, I would vomit. With each contraction, I would vomit. I just remember that the pain was unbearable. I was rushed to Florida Hospital and was admitted. At that time, I would become familiar with the word obstruction.

The doctor called my parents and told them to fly out at once; he said I would need surgery. But after all the IV pain meds and steroids, I felt better; enough to get released and go back to school.

The week after I was discharged, in 1990, is when I had my first colonoscopy. I drove myself there and drove myself home. I remember being groggy, but I felt okay to drive. (So young, so dumb.) I went back home and went into a dead sleep. My dad called me. He said, "Claude, you have Crohn's Disease." It didn't seem like a big deal.

I never thought of Crohn's as a significant problem. I was in my early 20s, motivated to make money, and Crohn's was the last thing on my list.

What I remember about that hospital visit was the pain. That never left me. Your first obstruction-related flare never will leave you. I wasn't fearful of Crohn's, I feared the pain and not getting relief.

COURT REPORTING AND A BABY

By the time I was 25, I had moved back to my home state, Rhode Island, and opened Merandi Court Reporting. I hired some of the best court reporters in the State of Rhode Island. Business was booming and so was my rectum. Owning my business, and working as a reporter, is when Crohn's made regular appearances.

I was sick, but it was my dirty little secret that no client could ever know. Nobody was to know that I was ill. I was a female business owner and people needed to know I was healthy and competent. My reporters knew I was sick, but they understood to never let clients know how sick I was. About five months after I met Francesca's dad, I needed to get rushed in. I couldn't stop vomiting and the pain was severe. The pain terrified me. Because I couldn't stop vomiting, they brought in the dreaded NG (nasogastric) tube. I despise the NG tube, but it brings relief instantly. It's a tube that goes up your nose and down your throat. While they were trying to put it in, I was fighting back. I remember seeing the back of my boyfriend's head as he was exiting the room. He couldn't watch the procedure. I heard him say, "This is gross." Right then, I knew this relationship could never work. He couldn't deal with illness.

One week after I was discharged, I found out I was pregnant. While I was in the hospital, I had one Remicade treatment and about 20 different medications during my hospital stay. My OB/GYN went through each record with a fine-toothed comb to see if any medication I was given would be harmful to the baby. He found one drug that could be of danger to the baby and that was Diflucan. It was used to treat a yeast infection. Francesca's dad and I broke off our relationship soon after I found out I was pregnant. I bought the house next door to my parents, who lived next door to my brother. (We're a little Italian). I was surrounded by my friends and family throughout my pregnancy, but it was a somber time for me.

I would try and keep a smile on my face, but I was devastated knowing I would be a single mom. I focused on my new home, my business, working as a reporter, and becoming a new mom. My parents were an integral part of my life during this time.

I gained close to 100 pounds during my pregnancy. I enjoyed every morsel of food I could find. I ate fried clams with the bellies and a gigantic cone of peanut butter cup ice cream nightly. I still trained at the gym, but dieting was out of the question.

My Francesca was born in July 2001, with my mom by my side. My mom was in the delivery room and brought her credit card and her Rosary beads. She stuffed them in her bra. Maybe she planned on buying an extra baby in the delivery room. I remember looking to my left because her scrubs slipped off and the anesthesiologist had to pull them up for her.

Francesca was delivered via C-section. She was four weeks early and was absolute perfection.

It was a bittersweet time. I had my beautiful baby, but I was also a single mom.

The stress came soon after I gave birth to Francesca. I had only seen her dad once throughout my pregnancy. His family visited but he didn't. I came out of remission in August of 2001. When Francesca was four months old, Francesca's dad demanded a paternity test. I felt like a whore; plain and simple.

My cross to bear in life was never Crohn's Disease or being a court reporter; my cross to bear was the custody battle I had ahead of me. But Crohn's gave me the will to fight harder. If it weren't for Crohn's, I wouldn't have survived what I would face over the next 14 years with custody dad.

CROHN'S AND MY PLUMBER

In 2003, I renovated my kitchen. I was running my business, raising Francesca, and having massive Crohn's attacks. It seemed like the perfect time to do a renovation. (I'm kidding.) I don't know what I was thinking. I needed to get admitted again. My dad would take care of my house, my mom would take care of the baby, and I would run the business from the hospital. Francesca's dad often traveled out of the country, so my mom would bring the baby everywhere she went. I had become a frequent flyer at the hospital. The cleaning people loved Francesca. Dietary staff would bring her treats, and she had every toy the gift shop could offer. After this hospital stay, I came home to a house under construction. One day I was rocking Francesca and I went in my kitchen. When I walked in, I saw someone under my sink. I asked, "Who are you?" He said, "I'm the plastic surgeon. I borrowed the plumber's tools." I hated him. I called my dad, crying, to come down.

I said, "Dad, the plumber is a fucking psychopath. Come down here." My dad said, "I like the guy."

Low and behold, Todd, (my plumber), and I started to date. When he showed up for our date, he had two bouquets of flowers: one for Francesca and one for me. I liked him, but I could never let him know what disease I had. I felt it was a disgusting disease. Men don't even want to think that their girlfriends poop, never mind what happens to a person with Crohn's Disease in the bathroom.

One night, he offered to take me to Sam's Wholesale Club. While we were driving, it happened. The rumbling started. I began to sweat. Todd was discussing something. All I remember was trying to focus on not pooping my pants. He kept talking and I was sweating and squeezing my hiney together. Christ, "shut the fuck up," I wanted to say. He's talking, talking; I'm squeezing, squeezing, and then that was it. I screamed, "SHUT UP!" He just stared at me. I cried, "I'm going to poop my pants." He got me to Sam's in under 10 seconds.

The secret was out. I told Todd everything. I knew he was my soulmate because the next day he said he'd been researching Crohn's Disease online.

He had me at, "Where's the shut-off valve?"

A BOWEL RESECTION AND A BABY

In 2003, the inevitable happened: I had my first bowel resection. It was a painful surgery. I was accustomed to pain, but this was a different pain. They needed to remove a small piece of colon, a good part of my small intestine, my appendix, and an old watch they found. (there was no watch.)

The recovery was hard. I went to the bathroom continuously. I remember looking at Francesca and crying. The pain, the diarrhea, the business, the legal problems with custody dad, my relationship with Todd, it weighed heavily on me. And I couldn't get back in remission. I developed wasting disease. I just got smaller and smaller every day. Food and water were out of the question. I was always in the bathroom. I had to get admitted again and again because of severe dehydration.

I was pissed because I thought this surgery would fix everything. It made things worse.

As the months progressed, I got accustomed to being sick and living in the bathroom. I called Todd one morning and told him I needed to go back in. When I was in the ER, I remember my lips were stuck together. If you pinched my skin, it would stay stuck together. My eyes were dry. I was severely dehydrated.

After the nurse hooked me up to fluids, steroids, and Dilaudid, the ER doctor came in. He looked so handsome, but everybody is beautiful when you're on Dilaudid. He said, "Ms. Merandi, you're pregnant." I disagreed with him. There was no way I could be pregnant because I didn't have sex. Todd walked in and told me to stop talking because they were calling psych down. Todd said, "Just disconnect her."

All I could think of is, "Oh, my God, my dad is going to kill me." I got knocked up, again, out of wedlock. That's all I could think of, was telling my dad.

My dad was so worried about me. It seemed like all he did was take me to the emergency room for fluids. The joint pain was debilitating. I was always thirsty. Now, telling him I was pregnant, I thought, for sure, this would kill him.

I was so sick. How could I be pregnant? But we had sex because I have a 12-year old in my kitchen as I write this paragraph.

We talked with the GI doctor. He told me I was too sick to carry a baby. He explained that I would go into remission, like I did with Francesca, but once the baby was born and those magical hormones left my body, I would get very sick. Many people with autoimmune illnesses go into remission when they're pregnant and I was one of them.

The doctor asked me to consider not having the baby. But that wasn't a possibility. Todd said that we would be fine.

16

When I was four weeks along in my pregnancy, I noticed I kept losing weight. I was diagnosed with hyperthyroidism. Every day I weighed myself, the scale dipped. I would die a little each day. We met with a doctor that specialized in high-risk pregnancies and she told me this was common. Things will improve by month four, but month four seemed like an eternity away. I wanted my baby so badly. I was deathly ill with morning sickness, Crohn's, and severe joint pain.

My mom and I took Francesca to an indoor amusement park. She was staring at Francesca. And I said, "Mom, do you like kids?" And she stopped and looked at me. She said, "Oh, God, he's going to kill me," meaning her husband, my dad.

We eventually shared the news. My father was devastated. He thinks I will die. He cries. I tell him it will be okay. I'm always telling people that it will be fine. All I have is faith in God.

Guess what? Month four, day one, I woke up and I wanted one thing: a pastrami sandwich with Doritos. I ate. A lot. I gained 17 pounds in one week. I used to set my alarm to eat. I would not miss one mouthful of food. I told Todd we needed to do an amniocentesis. What if I gave birth to something with horns on its head?

Todd was a wreck the day of the amniocentesis. The tip of the needle broke off while Ava was in utero, moving wildly. Todd almost fainted. But all was good, and Ava was healthy. Ava had been exposed to Remicade, so every kick was a welcome one.

On the day of my C-section, there were three surgeons, including a colorectal doctor, in the delivery room. I remember hearing Todd's breathing getting heavy. I was telling him how fine I was. Jesus, I'm always fine.

I heard the doctor say, "It's a girl!" Ava entered the world at almost nine pounds. Todd looked at her and he was crying. He said, "Babe, she looks like Francesca." And she had no horns. She was perfect. She looked tan, so she spent time under the lights. Once again, perfection. Not bad for a sick chick, huh?

CROHN'S, MY GIRLS, AND ONE SICK MOMMA

When I came home from the hospital with Ava, I got right back into the swing of things. There was no time to rest. I just had a C-section, but that was an easy surgery. I had to make sure everything with the business was running smoothly and I needed to spend quality time with Francesca. Francesca loved her new baby sister. I explained to Francesca all about nursing. Nursing, I was told, cuts down on the risk of Ava getting Crohn's by 50 percent.

We had latch-on parties in the hospital. It was hard to nurse, and I hated it. I remember watching all those YouTube videos, admiring all those calm granola-like mothers nursing their kid. They didn't swear either. They were really enjoying nursing. To me, it was like waterboarding.

There's pumps, creams, screams, and a baby who's constantly hungry. I ran to CVS one day. When I got back, my mom was holding both girls, waiting for me to nurse Ava. I swear to Christ, Ava knew when I was in the vicinity. She's five days old and I'm pretty sure she can smell me. Todd said, "Babe, you have to feed her." I stare at her. I'm afraid of her. She's big. "Are you sure she's hungry?" He said, "Babe, come on. Remember?

Crohn's?" I take a deep breath and hold it, hoping I'll pass out. I'm too embarrassed to nurse in front of people so I go in her room. Francesca follows. She said, "Mommy, what's that?" I said, "Francesca, honey, that's a crib. Babies sleep in it." I realized Francesca has been sleeping with my mom for four years. She's never seen a crib. I loved her sleeping with me or my mom.

Ava is staring at me and I'm staring at Ava. I'm trying to make a deal with a five-day-old baby. I think she's part bovine because she's always hungry. She latches on and I scream. Francesca, my little doll, giggles. Ava is eating like she's going to the electric chair. I'm fearful she's sucking the saline out of my implants.

At night, I started to run a fever. I kept it to myself. The night before, I had diarrhea eighteen times. I'm exhausted. Crohn's is back, and it wants its health back. I had red lines running from my breasts down to my incision. I made my way to my doctor. She said, "Take this and keep nursing." She gave me a script for an antibiotic.

When I got home, my dad is pleading with me to use formula. He notices I'm in the bathroom a lot. I went into Ava's room to nurse her. While I'm nursing her, I'm crying. I hear my dad scream, "Why is she doing this? Nobody does this anymore." My mom screams, "Billy, everyone does it now. They all nurse." Then my dad screams, "That's disgusting."

My parents are fighting about my tits and whether nursing is good or bad. I'm sweating. I screamed, "Shut the fuck up. This is supposed to be a peaceful time." My dad yells, "Claude, use the God-damned formula."

The next day, I had to get out to deliver transcripts. Clients wanted to see me. They all asked, "How are you?" "Oh, I'm great. Thank you for asking." On the way back, I stop to get Francesca a Happy Meal and die in their bathroom. I have Francesca sing, so I know she's okay. I need to see her feet under the stall while I'm on the toilet.

Francesca screams, "Mommy, you stink." Just keep singing, kid.

We get the Happy Meal and we made our way home.

The minute I walked in the door, Ava, the bovine, can hear my voice and wails. I go to nurse her and I noticed the pump was gone. I cried. I went in the kitchen. My mom said, "Daddy returned the pump. You're too sick." My parents prepared all the bottles. Ava gets her first bottle and she's content. She's happy. My dad is feeding Ava on one leg and has Francesca sitting on his other leg. There's calm. I'll take it.

Both girls were so beautiful. My dad would call Francesca, "papa." My father was over-the-moon in love with Francesca.

THE CROHN'S RETURNS WITH A VENGEANCE

Francesca started kindergarten, Ava is eight-months-old, and I'm back in the hospital. But before I go to the hospital, there's a whole routine to be completed before I "go in."

First, I lay out Francesca's uniform, piano lesson books, and favorite snacks. I rub Ava's "lovey" on me so it smells like me. I clean the house, get the reporters ready and then I can go. By this time in my Crohn's career, there's always a hospital bag packed.

When I get to the hospital, the doctor informs me the dead patient in the next room has more potassium than I do. My mouth is dry, my eyes are dry. I'm tired.

My mom or Todd bring both girls to visit. One girl is on each side of me in my hospital bed. I remember thinking, "I'm a burden to people."

The doctor came in and said, "I told you this was going to happen. You're sick. You need a bag."

"A Prada bag? I can't afford one." Get the fuck out of here. No bag, no way.

Legal woes were mounting with custody dad and I needed to hire an attorney.

With each legal issue would come another flare. It was a vicious cycle I couldn't control. But I was dealing with a man I couldn't reason with, partly because he works out of the state. But no matter how hard I tried, I could not communicate with this man.

As my girls got older, they both attended the best Catholic school close by. When I went in, everything had to be within five minutes of my home because my mom didn't drive on the highway.

My girls were always immaculate, punctual, and never missed one day of school or activities when I was in the hospital. Never.

Todd let me be a mother to Ava because I was the mom, but it was a different story with Francesca's dad. He needed to have the power. So, I would usually let him think he was the boss to pacify him. But things just worsened.

On the outside, things looked like a finely-tuned machine; the children, the business, the reporters, my relationship with Todd, everything seemed great. But things weren't great. Only my mom saw me sob at night. I was deathly afraid of losing Francesca in a court battle if I got sicker. I wasn't scared of death, I feared I would lose my baby. Bottom line: I couldn't get healthy. I was getting sicker by the day.

LINGUINE & CLAMS AND MY FIRST FISSURE

On Fridays during lent, I would make my family linguine and clams. It's a traditional Italian dish. Both my girls loved it. The 2011 Easter and Lenten season would be a memorable one for the family.

While my kids were feasting on their linguine, I was getting severe cramps that come with a Crohn's flare. They would make my mouth dry. Let the games begin!

Many people who suffer from Crohn's Disease describe the cramping as severe as labor contractions.

When I went to the bathroom, I felt a ripping sensation that took over my hiney. I screamed and screamed. I was holding on to the side of the vanity because this was a pain I had never experienced. Todd was banging on the door. The girls were asking, "Momma, can we come in?" I refused to look in the toilet because I knew Ed McMahon wasn't in there with a check.

No, God had a much different plan for me.

I turned around and my white tiled bathroom walls were splattered with bright, red blood. Ava was crying and wanted to come in the bathroom.

I screamed, "Don't come in." Too late. I looked to my left, and there's Ava, with linguine hanging out of her mouth while Francesca and Todd stared.

The pain was searing, and I knew whatever happened to my rectum was severe. I knew I had to go in.

I needed to clean the house and go through my whole routine before I went in. I had to clean the bathroom because it looked like a crime scene. I was in the bathroom and I could hear Ava screaming for me. I heard Todd telling Francesca to get my bag, and then I heard my mom's voice, "Honey, let me in so I can look." Since I was a kid, my mom always needed to see what's in the toilet. But now she's armed with a camera. I'm trying, desperately, to get things in order, while Ava is walking around with the linguine hanging out of her mouth while my mom is getting pictures. We're not calm people and it was chaotic at times.

Once I got to the ER, the doc insisted on doing a rectal exam. Absolutely, unequivocally not. He promised I wouldn't feel a thing with four milligrams of Dilaudid. He lied. He said I should be admitted.

Once I was admitted, everything was explained about fissures. Fissures are "special" because we get to relive the pain repeatedly until they're healed.

My hospitalist came in, and I couldn't understand what he was saying because of the language barrier. He's either from the Middle East or Maine. Because of all the Dilaudid, I just shake my head. He then explained why he doesn't agree with prescribing Dilaudid. Here we go.

I asked him if he wanted to play the "pick one" game with me. He didn't understand. I asked him to pick one of these conditions without Dilaudid. I gave him a choice of a fissure, fistula, kidney stone, bowel obstruction, NG tube, a catheter (that's an easy one, and it shouldn't even be included in the game) or a severe migraine with vomiting. He picked none. Sore loser.

The hospital priest, Father Eddy, walked in and the doctor asked him if he knew me. Father Eddy responds, "Claudia's the reason I chose celibacy." Father Eddy and I became good friends over the years while I was hospitalized.

I was first introduced to nitroglycerin cream when I got my first fissure. The minute you apply it to the infected area, your blood pressure drops, and you get a splitting headache. But this cream is better than Botox. Right around this hospital visit is when I would hear about the opiate epidemic and how they would stop prescribing Dilaudid.

THE CUSTODY BATTLE AND KIDNEY STONES

After I got home from my most recent hospital stays, I started my routine all over again. I checked on the girls, their homework, activities; then I switched over to the business and the reporters. I like to clean the house and throw out everything I can find. My mom takes the girls to the Dollar Store whenever I'm in the hospital and buys them twenty dollars' worth of shit. I go around the house with a black trash bag, so nobody can see what I throw away.

I've come to realize because I can't control my illness, I try and control everything else around me; house, kids, relationship, and business.

I was rocking Ava and Francesca and I could see my dad mowing the lawn for the second time that day. He then cleans the street and my driveway with the hose. I go bananas and scream out the window, "Dad, knock the shit off." My water bill is expensive, but my lawn looks pristine. If my neighbor's yard looked like shit, he would mow theirs. He believes it will increase the property value of his house.

I'm on a high dose of Prednisone and everything was setting me off. Francesca is playing with the deadly Polly Pocket toys. It's the toy my mother is convinced will be the death of my children because of a choking hazard.

While I was sitting in my chair, I got this jolting pain right in my lower back. I'm trying not to alarm the girls. But I'm crying because this is, yet again, a new experience. Francesca runs to get my dad. "Papa, papa, come in."

When my dad walks in my room, I'm on my floor, in my pink nightgown, and I'm vomiting and screaming simultaneously. I'm 'scromiting.'

"Claude, what's wrong?" "Dad, something's wrong."

He called the rescue. Oh, God, not the rescue.

I'm on the floor, rolling around, vomiting, holding my right lower back and I tinkled in my pants because I was vomiting with such force.

The rescue personnel arrive and are asking me questions. I recognize them because I am the court reporter for their arbitrations.

My first thought: they will see my big white panties. These are the comfortable panties that girls wear at home only.

I've lost all decorum. I know I must resemble women you see on that show "Cops."

I heard one firefighter say, "Hey, this is the court reporter." I'm mortified. The court reporter has tinkled her pants; and her nightgown, with the hole in it, is covered with vomit.

I can't even converse with them because the pain is something I've never experienced.

With Crohn's, there are so many pains, and they all suck.

Once again, I get admitted. The tests show seven kidney stones between my right and left side. They said that I was about to pass them. Pass them where, to my roommate, who's eating a Burrito in her hospital bed? I don't know what they're talking about.

The urologist tells me I must stay. But I can't. I just got released. I need to get back home. I can't keep doing this to my family.

But the pain that I'm going through with this illness is causing me to think differently. I told the doctor how I was feeling about having all this pain and my fear of it not being controlled. He said I was suffering from post-traumatic stress disorder.

CROHN'S AND A DYING PARENT

Francesca was six and Ava was two when my dad was diagnosed with stage four lung cancer. He as 71 at the time of his diagnosis. I knew he had cancer because he was grey. When my dad walked, he would wince. My father's life was my children. He had an extraordinary bond with Francesca. My family didn't want him to know what he had but I told him. The day my dad was diagnosed, I started to write his eulogy.

I used to take my dad for rides in the car. While we were on a car ride, he asked me what came after stage 4. I told him a coffin. We had a relationship where I could say things like that. He laughed and then he cried.

As the months progressed, it wasn't uncommon for my dad and me to be hospitalized simultaneously. By 2006, my Crohn's was labeled as severe. The hospitalizations depressed me.

My dad would ask me to read his eulogy to him. He would have me rewrite it and make it funnier. He adored Francesca, but he wasn't a huge fan of Ava's. He called her grumpy. Poor kid was always crying, wanting only me to hold her. Ava was very sick as a baby, but it leveled off when she was around 10 years old.

One night, Ava kept vomiting. She was one of those kids who couldn't stop vomiting. She would need an IV to rehydrate her, and anti-nausea medication to help her stop vomiting.

I had to take Ava to the ER one night, and I was exhausted. Todd and I would wait hours to be seen.

My dad was admitted the same day we took Ava to the emergency room. I was very sick and had to keep urinating while I was there. I had terrible pressure down there and assumed it was a kidney stone. But I was flaring. I remember thinking how exhausted I was.

Once Ava got in to be seen, I kept running in the bathroom. Only tiny amounts of urine would come out, but I was having severe diarrhea. Between waiting for the doctor, running upstairs to check on my dad, and getting the reporters' schedules figured out, I would be on the phone with my lawyer because we all had to meet the next day. Custody dad didn't want Francesca's tonsils removed. "For the love of Christ, when would this shit end," I thought to myself.

The stress of everything was taking a toll.

Once my dad lost his voice, we stopped all treatments. It was a hard decision, but we knew the end was near.

We would take turns giving him his morphine, as he chose to be home with Hospice. He picked out all his pictures for his wake, but he was fearful Ava would knock them down when she ran by them.

31

I read his eulogy to him, he reviewed his obituary, and his pictures were ready. He looked at me and said, "Claude, I'm sorry about your stomach." I said, "Dad, I'm fine." My dad was the funniest man I ever met, and although he was a complicated man to live with, he understood Crohn's. I went home to check on the girls. I was gone for five minutes.

My mom called me and told me to come back to the house. She said, "I think he died." I ran to their house, but he was gone.

My dad, William "Billy" P. Merandi lived a simple life. He was always writing letters to the editor, loved doing the New York Times crossword puzzles, and enjoyed the bathroom as much as I did. But his greatest joy in life was Francesca. He loved Ava but didn't get to know Ava.

The day after my dad was laid to rest, I had a massive kidney stone blasted. A one-day procedure turned into a seven-day hospital stay.

CROHN'S AND THE CUSTODY BATTLE

Francesca was nine Ava was four when we were embroiled in legal bullshit. Francesca's father's lawyer was an animal. He pursued this case with too much passion. The first lawyer demanded a paternity test, which was degrading, and his second lawyer was a fucking animal with an excellent reputation in court. Because I was a court reporter and a victim of the RI Family Court system, I trusted not one person.

I couldn't reason with custody dad or with his attorney. It was too much to handle. It was taking a toll on my health, on my family unit, and on my relationship with Todd.

It was always just my mom and me in the courtroom. My mother was exposed to so much. If she wasn't caring for me when I was in the hospital, she was caring for my children. Both dads worked, so my mom did everything.

But the court battle was scary. I didn't know what to expect. I just wanted to be a mother to my child, but custody dad had to have the last word. He had to have the power.

With each legal paper came a hospital stay; with each fight, came a hospital stay.

His prick lawyer thought nothing of it to serve me with papers while I was in the hospital.

The day we went to mediation, I told his lawyer that illness doesn't discriminate. He laughed and said I was crazy.... until he had his first stroke four weeks later. And there she was, that beautiful lady, that appeared before his prick lawyer; her name was Karma.

The minutia would continue with custody dad.

CROHN'S, FLU, PNEUMONIA, AND C-DIFF

In July of 2010, my accountant told me my business was getting audited. Great news. Right around this time, I was getting cramps in my stomach that weren't typical Crohn's-related cramps. Along with the cramping came massive amounts of watery, foul-smelling stool.

I'm in the bathroom thinking: the man I love will smell this. What the fuck is that smell?

My mom walked daily and would stop by on her walk. She walked into my house and said, "Ewww, what's that smell; did you cook broccoli?" It permeated the house.

I couldn't stop going to the bathroom, and I kept on bleaching the house. I was fearful one the girls would succumb to the smell. If you've had C-difficile, you know the smell. It never leaves you.

I got admitted the following day, and I tested positive for C-diff. I never heard of it until that day. When you have C-diff, it's the best and worst of hospital stays. You suffer from C-diff, but you get your own room because you're in isolation. C-diff stays colonized, so you don't know it's there. It's like when you're on a cruise ship, and the last day of the cruise you find a place and say, "Oh, man, I didn't know this was here." That's what C-diff is like, minus the onboard fun. It stays colonized, is what the doctor told me. It's highly contagious, so we assumed I picked it up in the hospital. While in the hospital, I was in contact with the reporters, with the girls' teachers, and with the business. Todd would keep the house immaculate when I went in. Todd was a stickler for Ava's hair to be perfect with a cute outfit on her when he visited.

My girls attended St. Luke's, which was a small, beautiful Catholic school. The school became a family. The teachers and principal would keep a watchful eye on my girls when I would go in. Ironically, two teachers at the school also suffered from Crohn's.

With each hospitalization, the tension would build between Todd and me. We both owned businesses, we were trying to raise three children, deal with the legal bullshit with custody dad, and battle Crohn's.

The tension would become greater between Todd and my mom. I felt torn because they both were my caretakers. She was my mom, and he was my fiancé. I was getting tired. I was getting sad. I wanted to please them both and be a great mom and be a great boss. But I was running out of fuel.

One night, after the girls were settled in for bed, I woke up confused. I was hot. I took my temperature and it was 105. I was rushed in. The nurses asked me if I was okay because I wasn't complaining. I didn't feel sick with Crohn's.

As soon as they read my temperature, I tested positive for flu and I went straight into isolation. My skin hurts. But the joint pain in my knees made me sob. I was crying and didn't know why. The pain was awful. Dilaudid did nothing for the pain. Tylenol was the only thing that worked. Three days into my flu stay, I developed pneumonia. I'm not a cougher. I rarely coughed. But I coughed so hard with pneumonia, I tinkled in my pants, and my port dipped down into my chest region. While all this was going on, my accountant was trying to contact me because the auditor had questions.

I was rushed into surgery. My port was removed and was replaced with a new one. All night, the wonderful nurses were trying, desperately, to access the new port. They couldn't make a connection, though. I remember this big, happy nurse with a kind smile, came into my room and said, "Honey, this may hurt." She pressed down, and I cried out. She accessed the new port.

I love having a port. When you're sick, the prick of the needle hurts even more.

I took four weeks to recover from pneumonia. I would continue to get the flu, yearly, for four years, even though I was vaccinated. Ava was a carrier for so many viruses. We nicknamed her Ava Ebola or Ava H1N1. The bottom line: my immune system was depleted. I guess that's why Crohn's is an auto-immune disease.

THE HOSPITAL ROOMMATES

By 2008, I had hospital visits down to a science. With Crohn's, the minute you wake up, you know if you're sick. For me, I would come out of remission during the night. 5 a.m. is the best time to go to the ER. It was "dead" at that hour.

Before I went in, I always had my bag packed. My "hospital bag" had my own toiletries, jammies, slippers, panties, socks, toothbrush, toothpaste, flat iron, Lavender scented room spray; but most importantly, a tweezer. Hair sprouts out on the face where it shouldn't while you're in the hospital.

I would kiss my girls goodbye at 4:30 a.m., lay out their uniforms and activity list for my mom. I always left at 4:30 a.m. because all the addicts had given up and went home, the workers' comp people don't arrive until 10 a.m., and whoever would have a heart attack or stroke usually did so by 2:00 a.m.

After going through all the bullshit in the ER, I usually was admitted and in a room in 12 hours from arrival time.

When transport would get me upstairs, everyone at the nurse's station would greet me. I was well known at my hospital because I was averaging about 60 days per year. They would inquire about my girls, my mom, and my hair. My hair always grabbed attention.

But then comes the dreaded time...that awful time when there's silence in your head. You're turning the corner to see which room you're going in and you start the praying game. "Please, God, let there be no roommate. If there is, please, let her be in a coma."

Now, if you're lucky, you'll test positive for C-diff and VRE. With C-diff, you can't get a roommate because you're in isolation. The nurse will try and sneak a C-diff in your room because there's a shortage of beds. But I'm no amateur. "Get her out," I would say. Plus, it's disgusting. When I have C-diff, I can't stand myself, never mind another person with it.

Once I would get settled in, I would meet my new lovely 400-pound roommate who farted so loudly and with such force she would blow holes through her panties. I usually got stuck with the roommate who had no social graces or would defecate all over the toilet and not flush. I would watch in horror when roommates would walk around with nothing on their feet or nothing on at all.

Or things could turn out differently, and I would get the sweet, old lady 89 years old, who also farts, but doesn't know she's farting. The elderly would call for aid to use the potty and it would take forever for someone to help them, so I would always offer help. Usually, they wouldn't make it in time, so they would tinkle and poop on my slippers, but it wasn't a big deal because hospital slippers were always thrown away.

What would irritate the shit out of me were the roommates that would have their 98 closest family and friends, who stay until 2 a.m. and they would binge on all stinky foods while I couldn't stop vomiting. They would laugh loudly, talk on their phones, EXTRA LOUD, until the wee hours of the morning and bring in stinky, deep fried foods. Those are the assholes.

I would call the nurse, and the nurse would say, "Claudia, they have rights, too."

So, on my way to the ladies' room, if they were awful roommates, I would throw a handful of glitter in their direction.

Then you had your roommates who would try and sneak their men in their bed while they performed various acts on each other. My mom one day asked, "What's that sucking sound?"

Last, my favorite roommates used the commode one foot away from me. I could hear them grunt, groan, curse and strain in various languages. We call this the "bowel movement language bank." That was always pleasant because there was a lingering odiferous scent in the room, a hospital room with no windows that opened. The lavender scented room spray came in handy.

THE DILAUDID

Throughout my younger years with Crohn's, I thought suffering was a part of life. I would hear my dad when he was in the bathroom, crying, so I just assumed I had to suffer like he did.

When I had my first massive obstruction, I was crying, vomiting. I knew if the suffering didn't stop, I couldn't fight anymore. When the pain becomes unbearable, you're rocking back and forth, praying to all the saints and it just fucks with your head. But then the nurse comes in, puts something in your pump and, bingo, instant relief.

Welcome to Dilaudid.

The nurse would say, "Honey, do you feel better?" "Yes, yes, yes." I feel better.

At 31, I lost my Dilaudid virginity. The suffering I would endure with Crohn's, kidney stones, and severe migraines would cause me to have suicidal thoughts. I hate writing those words, but I was always afraid of not getting out of pain.

By the time I made my way to the ER, I had waited at home for days, trying to self-medicate, so I didn't have to make the trip to the hospital. Nobody wants to go to the ER. When I get to the ER, I'm dehydrated, I'm in pain, I'm exhausted, and my only goal is to get out of misery. I need to be "still." That's the term that could best describe a person with Crohn's, who's been thrashing around in bed all night from the pain, running a fever and having severe diarrhea. It takes a toll on your body. And we all try and wait it out at home because if you go and you're not sick enough, you're sent home. So, you wait until you're on death's door to make the trip in.

But as I got older, I suffered no more.

The Dilaudid brings instant relief. Usually, my doctor would write an order for one milligram every three hours.

For me, Dilaudid and the telephone were a deadly weapon. Day two of a hospital stay, while on Dilaudid, I called my mom one morning. I told her that my furniture would be arriving at 10 a.m. and she had to be at my house to let them in. Then I would go into a dead sleep. She would call me screaming, "How much shit do they have you on? There's no furniture delivery." And then I would ask, "What furniture delivery?" That's Dilaudid.

Another time while on Dilaudid, I tried to get into the gift shop to buy a prom dress at 3 a.m. Or there was the time I made my way to the morgue, insisting I worked for a newspaper and was doing a local piece on death. Or there were the times I would call my clients, during the night, and sing the whole score from The Sound of Music, into their answering machine.

Dilaudid once cost me $5,000 while I was in the hospital. I booked an extravagant cruise for the girls and myself. Is Dilaudid a powerful drug? Most definitely. But to survive with Crohn's, Dilaudid is a necessity. Because I waited too long to go to the ER, it just made my illness worse and it extended my hospital stay.

During one of my hospital stays, I had a roommate, Mary, who just got her colostomy bag. I knew what she was going through. I felt for her. Her husband just kept talking about his workout at the gym. Mary just stared and cried. My heart broke for her. When her husband left, I asked her if she wanted me to file her divorce papers for her. She just stared. I said, "Mary, your bag needs to be changed." I could smell it. It was leaking. Mary had been waiting for the stoma nurse to get there. I told Mary I could help her. (this is a big no-no).

So, I shut the door, got her supplies laid out, cut her wafer (an ostomy supply), and I walked her through the steps of changing her bag. She was crying. I told her we would do it together and I would write down the steps for her. I told her to apply pressure to her stoma, so it didn't leak in my face. I wanted to make her smile because she was in hell. The first day with your stoma is hell.

First, I needed to give her a sponge bath because she hadn't showered in a few days. I laid out all my hospital supplies from home, washed her up, fixed her hair, and changed her nightgown.

When we were done, she smelled better and seemed to be in better spirits.

I fell asleep only to be woken by my colorectal surgeon telling me how much trouble I was in for helping a patient change their bag.

I had no recollection of changing a bag. That's Dilaudid.

When I was discharged from the hospital, I never took a script home. I was never offered one. When you're in severe pain, oral medication hurts. IV pain medication is what you need. And unless you're a doctor who's suffered from severe Crohn's Disease, we will agree to disagree.

THE COLOSTOMY BAG AND THE CUSTODY BATTLE

I'm in the hospital and the doctor comes in. He tells me, "You need a bag. Your body needs to rest. It will only be for six months." I've had thirty bowel movements in the past 24 hours and my potassium was a two. He tells me I'm at risk of having a heart attack. I tell him he's dramatic. My handsome surgeon tells me, "Claudia, you need to do this."

I tell them I couldn't have the surgery because I'm afraid I will lose custody of Francesca because I've been in the hospital so much.

Even though I'm a court reporter, I'm afraid of what could happen in family court. It's a dangerous place and anything could happen. My custody battle was a nightmare and navigating custody dad's mood swings were impossible. But I couldn't bear to keep running to the bathroom.

I went forward with the surgery.

When I woke up, I asked to see the bag. The nurse tells me there's no rush. My mom says, "Honey, not yet." But I needed to see it.

I look, then I sobbed, "I changed my mind, please reverse it, Please." I hear my mom crying.

After 30 days, I was released from the hospital. I was huge from the steroids. I was afraid to go home with the bag. I was on high doses of steroids. I felt so ugly. I felt so lost.

When I finally got home, I spent time with my girls, and I showed them the new addition to the family. I called the bag "whore." I watched every YouTube video I could find about changing the bag. But I realize quickly I'm not in control, the stoma is.

I was sitting in my chair, just staring, tears running down my face. I heard a knock on my door. I opened the door, and there stood a process server. The poor guy felt awful because he knew me. There they were, papers for custody of my daughter.

I collapsed. I sobbed. I called custody dad begging him not to do this. He told me I brought this on myself. I even called his girlfriend, but she didn't give a shit.

When Todd came home, he found me on the floor. I was lying on my side, in the fetal position, just weeping. Todd didn't know what to do. Nobody does. I kept thinking a judge would separate my girls because I was sick. How could this be? Custody dad doesn't even work in the state so how could he care for Francesca?

My best friend, Carole, showed up at my house with a care package. She knows I'm dying inside. She's been a court reporter for 30 years. She assures me everything will be fine. But she knows I'm breaking. I was trying to put a brave face on. She brings me gigantic panties, peppermint oil for the bag, and big stretchy pants. She notices the weight gain but says nothing. Carole is the friend who knew what to do because another friend of ours has a bag.

I remember thinking I wanted to die. But then I thought if I could eulogize my dad, I could get through this.

I had Francesca and her friends over to teach them how to make pizza the next day.

While all the sixth graders are stretching out their dough, Francesca says, "Mom," and she points to my neck. There's stool on my neck. The stoma leaked.

Both girls call my mom, "Nana, come here."

I tell the girls and my mom everything is fine. Everything is fine. I'm trying to get the wafer off but it's tearing my skin off. I assured my kids it's just like a band-aid and it doesn't hurt. They're trying to help, but my mom is panicking. I was panicking silently.

My mom and I went to the colorectal surgeon to meet with the stoma nurse. While we were waiting, we looked at the stoma. A mushroom came out. That was it for me. I gagged, and my mother gagged right along with me.

I ache for my mom because this custody battle is killing her because it's killing me because it's destroying our family.

It was my mom and me throughout this whole ordeal. My sister would have been there if she could, but that was it. Nobody could help. My dear friend was my attorney. She would assure me everything would be fine.

47

I have many friends and family that love me and were trying to show support, but nobody could give me peace of mind. There was no peace of mind. I was robbed of sleep, I was deprived of seeing my girls together. I was denied too much. People would call to check on me. But the words I would grow to despise were, "If you need anything, call me."

People don't know what to say to a chronically ill person. I, personally, would never ask a person for a glass of water, never mind a favor.

My advice: show up at someone's door with dinner, or walk their dog, or take their kids out for a few hours, but don't say those empty words.

Don't speak, just act.

THE 27 COLONOSCOPIES AND BEING A COURT REPORTER

As a court reporter, there are times in a deposition, hearing, courtroom, where's there's silence. And that's, usually, when you will hear my stomach at its loudest. I'm not hungry and I'm not in pain. That's just what a Crohn's stomach does. It's loud and sounds like underwater sea life.

Right before I had a colonoscopy planned, I got stuck doing a divorce case. I knew as soon as I saw the lawyers it would be a miserable day, and I was already not well. My job is to sit at that little machine, that you see on TV, and take down every word spoken. When attorneys fight, or people talk fast, I'll interrupt. This day, I had no energy.

We weren't on the record for 30 minutes before the attorneys fought over a Shalom plate. I'm trying to keep up, but I'm so dehydrated, my lips were stuck together. One attorney is objecting about objections and that's when I blacked out. I screamed, "Slow down. Holy shit. Jesus Christ." The attorney tells me I didn't look well. I was sweating profusely, and I was trying desperately not to have an accident. I couldn't control my diarrhea. But the fighting in this job was too much this day. At one point, I was asked to read back and I couldn't. I just stopped writing on the machine.

It was the first time in my career a deposition was suspended because of my Crohn's. I can't believe I lasted that long before it happened. The night of our annual work Christmas party, I had a colonoscopy done. I insisted on going. I was fighting to keep my eyes open while we were out. But I never wanted to let my staff down or my let my kids down because of Crohn's.

I've had over 20 colonoscopies and I consider myself to be a CCS, "Consultant Colonoscopy Specialist."

I had my first when I was a teenager. The way my mom described the prep, I knew she and my dad were lying and full of shit. I came home from school, and there it was: a gallon of white, murky-looking water. My mom said, "Honey, it's really not that bad." She's lying. But I remember how desperate they were to find answers because I was just getting sicker. Thirty-three years ago, it was straight Citrate Magnesium. Today, the bottles in the hospital say, "Ocean Prep."

My mom handed me the gallon. One sip. I vomit. Two sips. I vomit. My dad hears what's going on and I'm not about to mess around with a tired bus driver. "Claude, drink the shit." My mom holds my nose to get it down my throat. Now, they're both screaming, "Drink it. Drink the shit." My mom says, "Look, honey, mommy's drinking it." She gags. My dad is threatening bodily harm and my mom is screaming, "Billy, stop screaming at her."

I can't change my mind, again, because my dad took the day out of work to bring me.

Finally, after six hours, I get it all down. And then it begins; the urinating out of the rectum. And that goes on well into the morning.

The good news, the prep is completed. The unwelcome news: I have 25 more colonoscopies to look forward to.

The morning of my colonoscopy, when I was at my sickest, I was severely dehydrated. I felt awful. I wasn't up to doing the procedure, but I already completed the prep.

I was given the sedation drug they used, to no avail. I could hear the doctor talking, and with each turn of the scope, I could feel it and hear the gas being released into my stomach.

When I was wheeled into the "farting area," I said, "I want to see the doctor." The nurse said no, and I cut her off. "Now," I said. He came over. I asked him, "Why would you continue if you heard me screaming?" He said, "You weren't screaming, you were asleep." I said, "How come I know you had prime rib at the Capital Grille last night."

He stared. I stared. I was pissed. He said, "You're right. I'm sorry. We need to do them in the hospital with general anesthesia."

When you're inflamed, and you've been on pain meds for years, the sedation drug will not keep you comfortable. You will feel it. If you're a healthy person, you will be fine.

To this day, I can drink nothing that's clear except for water.

The last colonoscopy I had, I said, "Fuck it. I'm not doing the prep." I'd been admitted because I was having thirty bowel movements a day so what could be left? Plenty, because the doctor mentioned that I did an awful job with the prep. But the doctor could still maneuver through the contents of my stomach.

My advice: get the first appointment of the morning.

GOING ON DISABILITY

In 2005, my doctor came in my hospital room and told me to apply for disability. I did not understand what disability was. Between the stress of being a reporter, owning the business, raising my girls, and a looming custody battle, I caved, and I agreed.

I had to sell Merandi Court Reporting. I worked so hard at building my business and took such pride in knowing I had a great staff who liked being a part of Merandi Reporting. But one reporter gingerly explained I had a short fuse lately. She was right. I was tired. I was tired of being sick. The disability process is bullshit. It varies from state to state, with no reason given. Some people who had Crohn's for only two months get approved and then others with Crohn's for 30 years get denied. In Rhode Island, it's difficult. A handful of judges see the same cases again and again. And some judges just have NO on the mind. The process is flawed, and it needs to change.

I was denied after going through all the bullshit paperwork, not once, but twice. People would tell me, "Oh, you get it the third time." But why? What is the reason? I still don't know the reason. Why do you get it the third time or why do you not get it at all? I couldn't work as a court reporter and I couldn't work as a mattress tester. The process is flawed. I was applying for SSDI. I paid, into the system, from 14 until 40, uninterrupted. Was that the reason I was denied? Because they had to pay me too much money? I wish I knew the answer.

The third time I applied, I did it with an attorney, and he was phenomenal. We offered well over 800 records to the doctor that worked for Social Security.

The week before my hearing, I had a scar tissue surgery. That was, hands down, the most painful surgery I've had. But I couldn't miss my appointment.

My mom and I went together. We were waiting in this stinky area. Everybody that worked there looked disabled. All I remember is a woman with one leg, pacing back and forth, and with each pace, she farted, which made my mother laugh.

I was so tired from the surgery, but there was no way I would miss this hearing. I was embarrassed because I had a pillow held against my stomach, just in case I coughed.

When we were called in, I recognized the doctor testifying for Social Security. He read everything into the record. As he studied each hospital stay, each time I had C-diff, each surgery, I was fighting back the tears. The judge showed empathy and looked as dumbfounded as I was that I had been denied. The judge apologized and said, "This shouldn't have happened." And it shouldn't have happened. All those days I worked while I should have been resting, I blame on the process.

I was granted disability, and that would start the next chapter of my life.

And it wasn't a good one.

THE DEPRESSION

I'm alone during the day. I've dropped the kids off at school. I go home, and I crawl into bed. I stay in bed until 2:30, when I leave to pick up my girls from school. Todd moved out. I don't know if I blamed him or he blamed me. I have no idea. There was so much confusion in my mind. Todd is a good man, but he doesn't communicate. He would do anything for me if I asked, except for communicating. He treated Francesca as his own daughter. I look back at pictures of Todd holding Francesca with her pacifier in her mouth and I melt. But Todd didn't understand mental illness or depression. He thought I could just snap out of it. And I tried. God, I tried. Todd met a happy, spunky woman and he ended up with a girl that walked around the house in a bathrobe and an IV pole. But there was a dark hole I was stuck in.

My girls only saw a happy momma taking them to school and picking them up. Once I would drop them off, I would let "The Depression" set in. It was bad. Sometimes I would stare at a spot outside my window, sobbing in bed. I would be alone all day. I stopped eating, drinking, or trying to leave my bed while my girls were at school.

When I would wake the girls up, I would be happy. I would put on music on the way to school and then when I would drop them off, music went off. I went back to bed.

I stopped taking calls. I just let the phone ring. I would avoid my mom at all costs. I couldn't have people know I was depressed because I thought it was a sign of weakness. At least, I believed it was a sign of weakness. People were so accustomed to the girl who always rebounded, got right back into the swing of things when released from the hospital, and was always on the go. I stopped living. I was just existing.

I couldn't wait for the girls to get home. We would do homework, take their baths, and then I would have them both sleep with me.

I didn't want the morning to come. I just wanted it to stay dark. I just wanted my girls and me to stay in bed. Have it be nighttime all the time.

I would lie if I didn't consider suicide. But every time I thought of a plan, I thought somebody would get hurt. I knew enough to stop my mind from going to that very dark place.

I would ask Todd if we could try and work things out and he would block me out. It almost seemed cruel.

I went from not eating to always eating. Once I ate, I didn't stop. Ava would keep me company when I would open a bag of chips every night. Before I knew it, I packed on 30 pounds. But I was a shawl wearer, so you couldn't tell. No gym, no friends, no life. Just existing. The only place I went was to family court to battle it out with custody dad.

One day when I was in bed, I started to review the past in my mind. Did I really need to go to the hospital? Did I really need that surgery? Was I dramatic? Did I really need to stay all those days in the hospital? Was diarrhea really that bad that I needed to go to the hospital? Was the pain that bad?

Yes. It was all bad. I lost everything. Crohn's robbed me of everything. Depression comes with Crohn's Disease and many other chronic illnesses. It's real. And, sadly, too many people commit suicide because they just can't handle the physical pain or the mental pain. I prayed for guidance. I prayed and prayed.

One morning, I woke up. I looked in the mirror and said, "Listen, bitch, that's it. You're done feeling sorry for yourself." I knew if I was going to fight depression, I would have to help others.

I started delivering Meals on Wheels and I became an advocate for the elderly.

I lost my man, I lost my business, and I almost lost my daughter, but I could save myself. And that's what I did.

People don't like sick people. We're a nuisance. When you're sick, people disappear. They don't know what to say, how to respond, how to act.

And I don't blame friends or family for disappearing. But if we could bring awareness to the depression that comes with a chronic illness, then we're on to something big.

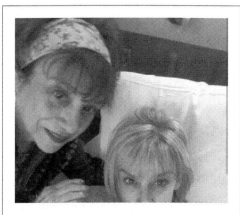

My Mom, always
at my bedside

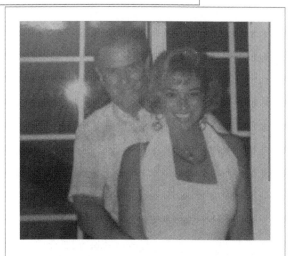

My Dad (1993) He
suffered from Chrohn's

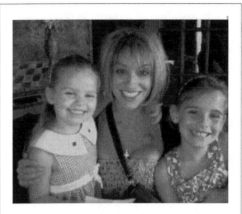

Momma and her girls

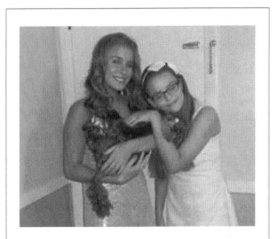

My favorite picture of my girls

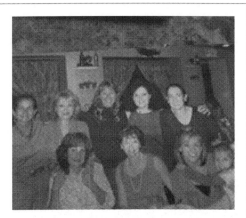

The Staff of Merandi
Reporting. Blessed to have
them

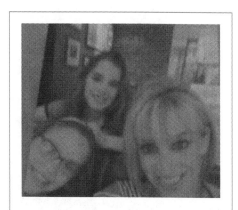

Me and my girls

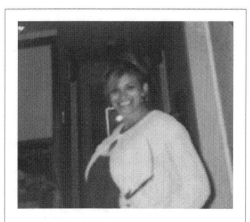

Pregnant with Francesca.
I gained 100 pounds!

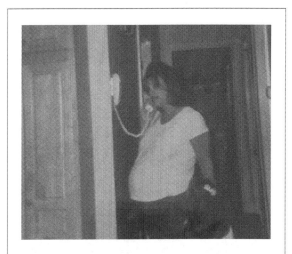

Pregnant with Ava,
another 100 pounds!

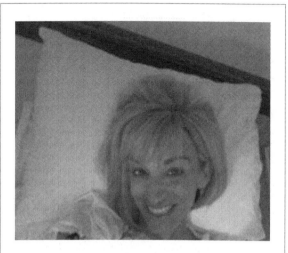

Back in the hospital

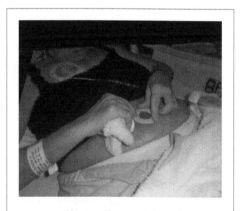

The dreaded colostomy bag day

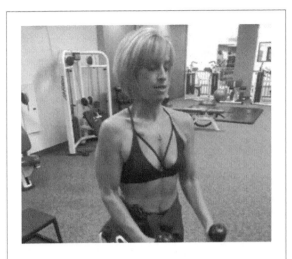

Transformation

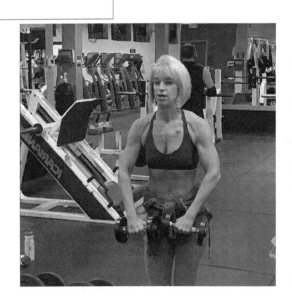

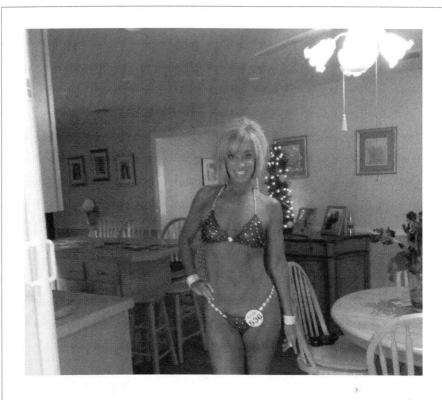

Taking Control of
my Life

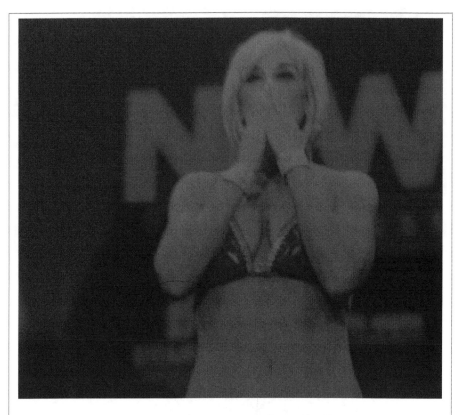

Set your mind and you
can accomplish miracles

TRYING TO LIVE LIFE

By 2015, I decided it was time to date. Dating was like a slice of hell. One was worse than the next.

Todd and I became so distant that I didn't recognize the man I once loved.

Ava hated that I wanted to date. She said, "Why date when you have me?" Ava knew I held onto the wish where maybe one day her dad and I would reconcile.

Prayer became an important part of my life. And every day, in those prayers, would be a special one that Todd would come back. I would see him nightly when he saw Ava, but he never looked at me. I would offer him dinner and he would decline.

We even vacationed together. That was great for both girls but not so great for me. Todd checked out, emotionally, while I was still checked in. I was feeling better. I trained again and ate healthy meals.

Dating was a disaster. I was dating people I wouldn't even have friendships with. I was acting desperate. I had longed for anyone to pay attention to me so when I met someone that showed me any attention, I thought I hit the jackpot. "Jack wrong." These guys were losers. As I look back, one was worse than the next. But it was something I had to get out of my system.

Eventually, I came to terms with being alone.

In January 2017, I pulled into my driveway, and Todd's truck was there. This seemed odd because Ava wasn't home.

I walked in and I asked him what was going on. He asked me to lay down next to him. My first thought was a boiler dropped on his head and he had a brain injury. But he assured me there was no industrial accident. He just wanted to talk. I didn't sit next to him because it seemed awkward. So much time had passed.

Once I talked with him, I knew what happened; the depression bug bit Todd. Work was a little slow and he woke up one day and felt tremendous guilt for leaving his family. I told him everything would be okay.

I just wanted him to know what I didn't know when I was depressed. He needed to know everything would be okay.

Todd came home. My prayers were answered. Todd, Claudia, Francesca, and Ava were a family again. I felt like it was Christmas.

But a few things changed since Todd left. I reinvented myself, and I discovered my worth. It took years to do, but I achieved it.

Everything was terrific for three months. I was just so happy to have Todd back home. That's where he belonged.

Unfortunately, it was short lived. For the people that followed my blog, there wasn't the happy ending we all expected.

Todd left in October of 2017. He just wasn't in a place to be in a relationship. And I don't think he ever was. In hindsight, we didn't have much in common. But I so desperately wanted Ava to have the family unit. Francesca was put in an awful situation, but Todd didn't have the hatred in his heart like custody dad. Todd wasn't like that. Todd was happy knowing Ava was happy and Ava was happy being with her momma. But this time, I knew I did everything I could do to make Todd happy. I was okay with him leaving. Some people just don't belong with a partner. That could be me or that could be Todd.

But I was healthy, training hard, and putting all my energies into making up for lost time with my children.

I will always love Todd. I will always not love Todd. It's just one of those things.

Todd trusted my judgment and he knew everything I did for Ava was good for Ava. Even when I was in the hospital, I knew the right thing to do for Ava. Education, doctors, tennis, playdates, I made all the decisions. And because Todd let me be a mother to Ava, Ava is a very happy little girl. Custody dad robbed me of all those beautiful experiences I was able to share with Ava.

I love my plumber, but I guess he wasn't my soulmate. And some days that makes me sad. I knew Todd needed to leave because I started to flare. I love Todd, but I love me more.

THE DREADED ER VISITS

In 2013, I was in and out of the hospital every three weeks. I just couldn't get into remission. I spent one last night in misery before I went in. Going to the ER could be a good thing or a terrible thing. And with the opiate epidemic at its height, you were always flagged as a drug seeker if you were a frequent flyer.

It was a Sunday morning, and the place was dead (no pun intended.) I was taken in right away.

As soon as my nurse walked in, I was screwed. The only nurse in the entire hospital I didn't care for walked in. She was the type that wore too much makeup, had lipstick on her teeth, desperate to marry a doctor. She said, "What, now, Claudia? Ugh… you have a port?"

And here we go. I'm already sick and Morticia wants to challenge me. I asked "Tish" if accessing my port would be a challenge. "Ugh…it takes forever to find the needle." She's usually hateful, but today she was extra repulsive.

She accessed my port and the doctor came in. This doctor had treated me at least fifteen times in that past, including admitting me. He was cold. He was acting differently. Something was off in this ER.

We are officially in the throes of a dreaded ER visit.

I explained how I was feeling, my symptoms. I was having severe joint pain and the usual Crohn's symptoms.

The nurse came back in, put something in my port that I wasn't familiar with, and said, "You're all set. We're releasing you." I disagreed. The nurse said, "Look, you're not getting pain meds because we're all being monitored."

I told her that was unacceptable and that I would gladly wait for the next ER doc. I was crying. I was in a surreal situation. I told her no way would she de-access my port only to re-access it. I knew something was wrong with me Crohn's-wise.

The chief nurse came out. I've never seen this man in my life. His breath smelled like rotten eggs and he was making me sicker. He oversaw all the nurses and he seemed like he hated his job and I was just making his life hell, I'm sure.

By this time my mom had arrived. I was crying.

I waited to see the next ER doc. His first words were, "You're going through withdrawals." My mom asked from what? I was released three weeks ago. I told the doctor that was nonsense.

Now everybody in the ER knew the situation. It was a slow Monday morning. A new nurse came in and did a flu test. She was so rough. My mom said, "How dare you be so rough with her?" The nurse said not a word. The doctor came back in and said, "I just spoke with your GI, and he said you no longer have Crohn's. There's no reason for you to be

here." I was confused. I was crying. I was humiliated. The doctor came back and said, "Your flu test was inconclusive, so you don't have it."
I had enough. I said, "Mom, let's go."

My mother attacked the doctor, told him he had no compassion, and we were filing a complaint.

When I got home, I crawled back into bed. I had been robbed of my dignity and I was just getting sicker. But there was no way these two doctors would walk away from this incident unscathed.

The next day, I received a phone from the hospital telling me I tested positive for the flu.

I was getting sicker and I started to bleed.

What was I going to do? Where was I going to go? Who could help me?

I made a vow: Nobody would ever treat me like that again. And if they do, I'm going after their license. I also vowed to help others that would soon experience this same treatment in hospitals nationwide. This is the hospital that my Blue Cross paid 9 million dollars to over 30 years. This is the same hospital that always showed me compassion. But things were different now.

Over my dead fucking body would this happen to me again.

THE AFTERMATH OF THE BAD ER VISIT

After I was released from the ER, I composed many letters to different people. I sent one to the Chief of the ER, the Department of Health, and one to the Editor of the Providence Journal.

I was getting sicker each day. I called my GI and explained the situation. Between custody dad, the severe joint pain and constant trips to the bathroom, my GI told me to go back to the ER.

Once I arrived, I was treated with compassion and admitted within the hour. I explained the circumstances surrounding my last ER visit to the ER doc I saw this day. I wanted everything to be documented. I made sure my mom was with me and I would record every word spoken. I wasn't taking any chances.

Once I was in a room, the doctor came in and said my SED rate was high and I was bleeding, something which I hadn't experienced, except for a fissure. But this pain was deep in my stomach. I was back on IV Dilaudid, large doses of IV steroids, Cipro, Flagyl, and potassium. My doctor suggested a colonoscopy. I said, "Wait a minute. You told the ER doc I

73

was healed and no longer had Crohn's." He said, "I never talked to the ER doc. You should have been admitted."

My mom and I were disgusted with the last ER doc situation, but I needed to prep for the scope. The other matter would wait.

I tried to get the prep down. I drank it all and vomited it all. Prep was out of the question.

The next morning, I was brought down. I recognized all the nurses and we were talking about our kids because they went to the same school. I was given "Milk of Amnesia" and went into a deep sleep.

When I woke up, I needed to use the restroom. The nurse told me no. I said, "I have to go." She said, "No, you just think you have to go." I had an accident everywhere. I knew my body well enough. Having an accident is humiliating.

Once I was wheeled up to my room, the doctor and my mom were there. They were silent. My mom looked like she was crying.

I said, "What's wrong?" My doctor said, "Claudia, your Crohn's has spread, there are lesions, and there's a layer of Colitis you haven't had before. It looks pretty bad."

All I could think of was the ER doc who said I was cured. Cured?

After the doctor left, my mom and I made our way down to the ER to find that doctor. To my surprise, he was there. I said, "Do you remember me? I'm the girl who was cured of Crohn's. Read this." My mom told him one day he would have kids of his own and to pray they're healthy.

74

And this, my friends, is how an ER visit could cost you your life. You always need another person when you go to the ER. If you're being treated unkindly, record everything.

The opiate epidemic has doctors on high alert and I understand that they're being policed. But you cannot discount the entire chronic illness community because of the opiate epidemic. Millions suffer from chronic illnesses and to paint us all with the same brush can cost one their life. My mom said, "You should get a bill passed." One day on Facebook, I posted the logo for "THE ER COMPASSION BILL FOR THE CHRONIC ILLNESS COMMUNITY." The response was overwhelming. Not hundreds, but thousands of others were going through the same thing I was going through. How could this be? If we can't get pain meds from our primary care doctors or our GI doctors, where we would go to treat our pain? If this continues, the chronic illness community will be seeking relief on the streets.

 When I would go to the ER, it was because I needed IV pain medication. But now the ER couldn't offer me relief because of the opiate epidemic. If you had an addiction, you could go to a clinic and receive treatment but if you suffered from a chronic illness, you were screwed.

My PCP introduced me to a pain clinic in Massachusetts. My doctor was an anesthesiologist. We finally found a daily pain medication that would give me my life back. I didn't like taking pain medication daily, but it was better than living in a hospital bed. Before pain management was introduced into my life, I was existing. That's all I was doing. Now, I'm living for a cause. But why wasn't pain management mentioned to me before? Why wouldn't one of my doctors suggest this? It makes one wonder.

(My representative will be endorsing and sponsoring THE ER COMPASSION BILL FOR THE CHRONIC ILLNESS COMMUNITY IN JANUARY 2018.)

My goal: When you enter an emergency room, there will be the logo of the bill, and it will say, "This hospital recognizes the chronic illness community and we strive to treat all patients with compassion." That's all I'm looking for.

If we could pass this bill in the smallest state in the union, Rhode Island, it could trickle into the other states. It wouldn't dictate how a doctor could practice, but it would bring attention to "our" epidemic.

THE HOSPITALISTS

For most of my Crohn's career, I was fortunate to have my GI doctor admit me. I sent a letter to the Chief of Hospitalists explaining why it made more sense to have a doctor, who knew my illness, who has been treating me for this specific disease, admit me and put in my orders. I'm not a fan of the hospitalists. There may be good ones, but I wasn't impressed. They seem to be a jack of all trades, master of none. And living in a hospital bed for many years, I saw everything and anything imaginable.

When I was admitted in 2012, I was greeted by a small, white lady, who appeared to be a doctor. She looked 14 years old. She came in chewing gum with both her hands in her pocket. She introduced herself and asked, "What brings you here today?"

"I didn't have any plans and I was craving hospital food."

I explained to her what was going on and she nodded her head, while both hands stayed in her pockets. We stared at one another. She said, "Well, I just want to tell you that I won't be giving you any IV pain meds."

Check, please.

"And take your hands out of your pocket when you meet your patient. You're not twelve. Show some respect."

I was admitted and released in four hours.

What I needed that visit was IV steroids because the joint pain was unbearable. But I left. I was too sick to fight with someone who was a doctor for less than a year.

I called my pain management doctor, who's also an anesthesiologist, and he told me he was continuously receiving phone calls from other patients from various hospitals in Rhode Island.

Over the next few days, I would continue to get sicker.

The inevitable happened and I was going to be readmitted.

I dreaded getting wheeled upstairs. I was stressing about the stress that was about to go down with another hospitalist.

When I met this doctor, he assured me he had treated others with Crohn's, but I wasn't convinced. He seemed a little flighty, a little confused. He was a moron. He was a doctor who belonged in a walk-in facility.

Now, the hospitalist is supposed to work with and confer with your treating physician, your GI doctor, and they SHOULD, together, come up with a plan. Now, if you get a hospitalist, who's had experience, some common sense, he'll usually heed advice from the doctor that's been treating you, in this same hospital, for over 20 years. But you could get a cocky hospitalist who wants to save the world and then we have a pissing contest.

A hospitalist does not want to be dictated to by a real doctor -- I mean a doctor that specializes in certain fields. And if you're offended by that comment, you're a hospitalist.

I had been admitted to only one hospital in my life and spent hundreds of days there. I had all my surgeries performed there and all my records were in one location. Why on earth wouldn't the hospitalist, take some time, look at my file for the past 20 years, and treat me with what I had been receiving and what worked? Because they're fearful of losing their license or getting written up. That's why.

Nighttime rolled around, and my pain was severe. I'm thrashing around, grabbing the rails. My male nurse came in and said, "This is bullshit. Your blood pressure is off the charts. You need pain medication."

This son-of-a-bitch hospitalist would not agree with my GI doc about the pain med situation.

I was finally given something after the male nurse called the on-call hospitalist.

The next morning, I awoke to find my GI doc sitting in the chair next to my bed. He said, "I think you have PTSD."

When you have suffered your whole life with Crohn's and you're in pain, you're rocking back and forth, you try the fetal position, the heating pads, the sweating, the crying, the shitting of the pants, of course you're going to suffer from post-traumatic stress disorder. I always remember my first blockage and being in severe pain and then getting out of pain. That first blockage never left me. And my fears would grow, at home, knowing I may or may not be treated when I would get to the hospital.

Day three, my fever spiked, my blood pressure was up, white blood count is up, SED rate is high, and I'm going to the bathroom five times an hour. That's it. I'm done. I called Risk Management. My mother, who was in her late 70's said, "But what is going on here? This is a hospital. She's going to die." No way would my mother sit back another minute.

I summoned Risk Management, and before you know it, Larry, Moe, and Curly, all three hospitalists, are in the room with two people from Risk Management along with my GI doc. They were all about to get a dose of my mom, Dotty Merandi. I pitied them. My mother doesn't fuck around. She's been living in a hospital, with me, since I was a teen. How much of this nonsense must we take? When is enough, enough? When you're dead?

Larry, Moe, and Curly wouldn't take accountability for their negligence, and I had my lawyer on the phone. Risk Management said that that wouldn't be necessary and just like that, I was on IV steroids, Zofran, potassium, Cipro, and one milligram of IV Dilaudid every three hours. Look what I had to go through to receive treatment.

Had the hospitalist listened to my GI doc, who's been treating me for over 20 years, this all could have been avoided. But why do we have to go through all these machinations to get pain relief? How does the opiate epidemic involve a person who's been living with an illness for their whole life? We're accustomed to pain and we're accustomed to pain medication. Knock the shit off and treat your patient with the compassion and dignity they deserve.

I take notes every time I'm admitted, even if a situation doesn't concern me. I refuse to watch somebody treated without dignity.

AND THE BULLSHIT ER VISITS CONTINUE

In March of 2017, I hadn't been feeling well for at least a week. At night, I would feel worse and would pray for relief by morning. My mom kept telling me to go to the ER. I couldn't put myself through this. Just the thought of entering the ER would bring on anxiety. This is how bad the ER visits had become. And I would speak with hundreds of others who would endure this type of anxiety when making a trip to the ER. I would prepare myself for "the interrogation" if I went in.

But I had to go. I couldn't take the pain any longer. When I arrived at the ER, it was 5 a.m. on Sunday. That's usually a safe time to go.

The nurse who came in was pleasant and accessed my port with ease. When the doctor came in, I told him I was flaring and that I also felt a fullness in my bladder. I told him I was nauseous and that the pain was terrible. He inquired about the pain meds I was taking at home. Here we go. I explained to him that I was having breakthrough pain. I told him I felt out of sorts. I really couldn't explain it better than that. He asked me, "What do you want me to do for you?" I turned my phone on.

I reiterated to the "doctor" my symptoms. He stared. I stared.

He told me he would call my GI doctor. I could hear him on the phone, laughing. I heard him say loud and clear, "I'm not giving her Dilaudid." Once he came back in the room, I told him I was recording him. I said I heard his loud conversation. I asked him for anti-nausea meds. He said, "Here, this works better." He ripped open an alcohol swab and told me to smell it.

As he was walking away, I asked him if I could talk with him. He said he was too busy and he would "throw" it over to the next doctor.

I called my mom. I was crying but not shocked. We knew this would happen.

Two days later, the pain was severe. I went to the urologist's office because I felt pressure in my vagina. In less than two minutes, the technician told me I had a huge stone blocking my kidney. The urologist couldn't understand how the ER doc could miss this. She said I needed surgery. I was afraid to go in because I just had Remicade. I waited another 24 hours but couldn't wait another minute longer.

When I reluctantly, returned to the ER, the red carpet was rolled out. I was terrified to return to the ER again. I assumed I would be treated unkindly. But just the opposite happened.

The ER doc came in. He said, "I'm sorry about what happened a few days ago. I'm going to make sure you're comfortable until you go to surgery." And just like, I was out of pain. One doctor, a hateful prick, who already had a preconceived notion I was a drug seeker, and now you have a doctor who's compassionate. I just don't understand how two doctors could have such different opinions, yet work in the same field, in the same ER.

I had the kidney stone blasted and woke up with a stent. I never had a stent before. I was miserable. The pain was awful. Four days later, I had the stent removed. There was no way I would have the stent taken out in the doctor's office. I know millions of people do, but I chose not to. No, thanks.

I was fed up. So, I wrote my letters. I wrote one to the editor, one to the Chief of the ER, and this time, one to the Senator's office.

Many who suffer from Crohn's also have the pleasure of enjoying kidney stones. It's due to malabsorption.

One simple renal x-ray could have prevented this. One x-ray. But one tired doctor couldn't, or wouldn't, go the extra mile.

The next time I return to the ER, it will be when my bill has been passed.

CROHN'S AND "THE SEX"

When I blogged about sex, it became known as "THE SEX BLOG." I knew when I wrote this specific blog, it would be descriptive. I needed to write things that people wanted to discuss on the support groups but were embarrassed to do so. So, when I wrote it, I went full throttle. I have Crohn's Disease but I still like sex. But sex and Crohn's/UC can be tricky. My biggest fear about writing this blog was that my mom would read it. Having sex in my 20's and living with Crohn's, never presented a problem. I had more sex thirty years ago than I do now.

When I met Todd, I fell madly in love with him. I wanted to make him happy in the kitchen and the bedroom. He knew I was sick, but the poor bastard had no idea what he was in for.

Let's face it: the first year of any relationship consists of two things: going out to dinner and having sex.

But after my bowel resection, keeping water down was a challenge. But I always led Todd to believe that I was okay. I didn't want him to know about my regular bathroom habits. We would go out to dinner, and I would play around with my food because I knew we would have sex later in the night.

Now, eating and having sex in one night is a highly dangerous situation. It's one or the other. Both in the same evening rarely happens. I would suggest having sex before dinner. But nobody likes sex or dinner at 3:30 in the afternoon.

One night I got all dressed up, and my mom had Francesca for the evening. This would be the night I rocked his world. We had planned a romantic dinner. So, I, to prepare for my sex night, took six Lomotil, one Vicodin, and three Imodium. A stick of dynamite couldn't penetrate my colon. This would be known as the S, C & F night: sucking, clucking, and fucking night. It was anything but that.

He chose a restaurant that was the home of the three-pound baked stuffed lobster. I was screwed. We sat down, and the smell alone was making me nauseous or it could have been the cocktail of drugs I took earlier in the day. When they brought out our dinner, I looked at the food, and I could hear my stomach rumble.

I ate nothing all day, I worked out, my hair was perfect, and I had on a little slutty outfit. My stomach was so loud that Todd asked, "Is that your stomach?" "Who, me? No."

After dinner, we made our way back to his house for "the sex." My mother calls sex, "the sex."

Now, ladies with Crohn's have different struggles than ladies without Crohn's. First, we worry about the vaginal sounds that sneak out during sex, but with Crohn's, we were dealt a double whammy; what sounds will escape from the rectum and the vagina? I always offered to do other things instead of "the sex."

I blasted the music. If I remember correctly, Norah Jones came on or The Wiggles. We both had kids around the same age, so The Wiggles was a definite possibility.

I was really into Todd, but my stomach wasn't, and my ureter wasn't either. Every time we would have sex, I would get a UTI. This, again, seemed to be common with other ladies I knew who suffered from autoimmune diseases.

When I would get a UTI, I would get confused, high fevers, and before you know it, the UTI would cause me to flare.

Todd would always ask if I was okay because the stomach sounds were hard to differentiate from the sounds you would hear at SeaWorld.

When I would have sex, the thought was always there: am I going to have an accident? My legs are wide open, so anything is game. With Crohn's, you never want to have anything wide open. The hiney has a mind of its own and accidents are frequent.

I would pray, "Please, God, don't let me have an accident on my plumber."

The "sex night" was a disaster. My head was pounding from all the Lomotil and I was starving. But Todd was sleeping over and I couldn't chance the unknown.

Todd wanted to have pillow talk, but I was hallucinating about suffocating him with the pillow because I felt so sick.

A few weeks after, I came clean and told Todd everything about how Crohn's and sex sometimes present problems. I said I would understand if he didn't want to date but he didn't seem to mind.

But sex and Crohn's would prove to be a challenge. Todd was afraid to have sex because of me getting a UTI, which would cause a flare, which would lead to a hospital stay. We were both self-employed and time was money.

I'm 49 now but I know one day, my Knight in Shining Armor will arrive at my door and we're going to have amazing sex. I just hope I still have my teeth and hearing when he shows up.

CROHN'S AND STRESS

If your doctor tells you stress does not worsen Crohn's, he/she is full of shit.

Stress is just as deadly as an obstruction to a person with Crohn's. You stress, you flare; you flare, you go in.

When I was going through my custody battle, if I saw custody dad's number pop up on my phone or see his car in the school parking lot, my heart would drop. You could hear my stomach rumble. That's stress.

Trying to control your stress when you have diarrhea running down your leg is impossible. But stress is part of life. Add a few teenagers in there, a full-time job, a spouse, some renovations to the house, a few financial woes, and you're good to go... straight to the hospital.

When stress started the de-remission process, I would feel like a failure. I would feel like I let everybody down. When I would walk into the ER, it felt as though I was doing the walk of shame.

How fucking crazy is this thinking? I've been up all night, having severe diarrhea, unbearable joint pain, yet I feel guilty about going in because I let "custody dad," once again get under my skin.

If you're a woman, you were raised to feel guilty if you do not please the entire universe.

For most of you Warriors, the stress could start at work.

If you keep running to the bathroom. Stress.

Your boss is giving you the evil eye because you spend too much time in the bathroom. More stress.

You fantasize about removing your teenager's vocal cords because you two are at each other's throats. Stress.

Or you're worried you will lose custody of your child because you're in the hospital again. Stress.

You're up all night in the bathroom because your mind nor your rectum will shut down and before you know it, you're in a full-blown Crohn's flare. Your rectum is on fire because you can't stop going to the bathroom and then you have heating pads everywhere, but you're fearful you'll catch on fire if you sleep with three going at once.

This is called Crohn's-induced stress.

But I have good news for you: you can pick your stress. For me, custody dad was my biggest stressor, so I needed to end that. I stopped all contact with him. My daughter is a good kid and she was old enough to communicate on her own. She benefits from her dad and I no longer speaking. But that's okay. I'd take my chances if it reduced the stress. And we would all be happier for it.

The second thing that needed to go: all negative people; friends and family included. My mom is 82 and looks at the negative in a situation before it even occurs. She's a genetic warrior. She worries about worrying when there's nothing to worry about. But that's okay. I'm not a worrier. I gave it up to God years ago. I figured if I couldn't handle the situation on earth, then God would take it over. And He has never let me down.

Once I cut all the assholes in my life, I reduced my stress. Now, this sounds like a straightforward process, but it took years to perfect.

Once I was able to cut the stress I could also control the flares.

To be realistic; we can't end all stress. But the issues that caused me to flare, I could discard. And that's what I did.

As a person who's suffered from Crohn's for many years, I never believed that stress or food could worsen my illness.

I was never so wrong about anything in my life.

CROHN'S, FITNESS, AND MY TRANSFORMATION

When I wrote this chapter, it was two years ago that my mom's identical twin had passed. My mom was devastated. She felt as though she lost a limb. I needed to lift her spirits. My mom is my best friend, my biggest fan, my caretaker, my children's' mom, and my heartbeat. Without my mom, my chances of survival were slim to none.

We were in the car one day, and I said, "Mom, I think I'll do a show in auntie's memory." She asked what kind of show, and I told her, "A one-woman play about a girl who got knocked up twice out of wedlock." She didn't think like that idea. "Mom, a fitness show."

She loved the idea. Instantly, she was on board. I always admired the girls in shows, but there was one thing stopping me: I was chubby. I put on a layer of love because I had been in remission for a year and I enjoyed eating again.

I have always been a gym rat, but being a fitness competitor was on a whole new level. I called my old friend, Kevin, who I trained with years earlier. Kevin was well known throughout the state and had an excellent reputation. When I met with Kevin, I told him I wanted to create the best body I could create without dying or coming out of remission. I trusted him. He's a gentle soul, and the promoter of the show I would enter. Kevin knew my health issues and knew how sick I was. He created a diet and workout regimen for me, and he said, "We'll see how far we can go. If you get sick, you don't compete."

Game on!!

Now, three things had to be eliminated right from the beginning: bread, pasta, and all negative people.

As Kevin measured me, I noticed all the beautiful women on posters who had competed. None had scars from colostomy bags or multiple incisions. There were no saggy knees, no cellulite, and they all had amazing asses. I had my breast implants removed, so I didn't even have that going for me. I had my breast implants removed out of desperation. I thought a foreign body could be causing my body harm and wreaking havoc on my Crohn's. When I was looking at those posters, I said, "I'll never look like them." I mean these girls come from a sick gene pool and most are healthy.

Kevin created a diet and a training program. He would quiz me about what a meal is, a snack meal...all the essentials to lose weight. The hardest part of this diet was drinking one gallon of water daily. Everything that I ate was prepared only by me. When I went out to dinner, I packed my baked sweet potato and my steamed broccoli. It seems it's a burden for a restaurant to steam broccoli. I would only order grilled chicken. I told the waiter to have the chef wipe down the grill. With Crohn's, I could not tolerate the smallest taste of butter. And

93

everything that is made in a restaurant starts with two ingredients: butter and olive oil.

When we would go to family gatherings, if somebody offered me something, my mom would say, "She can't eat that. She's doing a show." I did one hour of cardio every day, even though I was supposed to take a day off. Every day I would train a different body part.

When I was three weeks into the process, I posted on Facebook I would be competing in my first show. The support I received was overwhelming. Mostly, on Facebook, you would see me in a hospital bed. Every day, friends and people I didn't know would post inspirational words. It gave me something to look forward to. I had a purpose. It felt like a full-time job.

But there was one barrier; I never wore a bathing suit in public. I never wore a bikini. I didn't even own one. The thought of wearing one would keep me awake at night.

Week five into the process, a trainer at the gym, Josh, came up to me and asked me if I was doing a show. I was astounded. Did I look different to others? Eventually, Josh would become my trainer for my second show and help me on days that I would train legs.

Leg days would always bring me out of remission. I would get sick. Josh knew about my health issues, so we took it slow.

But the bikini process was a daunting one. My mom and I met with my bikini seamstress, Roanne. The first time I put it on I cried. All I could see was cellulite and no ass. "Oh, my God, I can't do this," I thought. I was getting anxious.

The next day, I would work even harder at the gym. Roanne would say, "You're six weeks out. That's a long time away." Six weeks out means six weeks away from the show.

My mom was horrified when I came out with the bikini. She said, "Oh, my God, I can see your vagina. Oh, no, it needs to be bigger."

Roanne said, "Absolutely not. Her ass will look bigger with a bigger suit." After every fitting, I would push harder and harder.

Learning to pose was a necessity. When I went to the posing class, I discovered there was a transformation category. This category was for people who lost a massive amount of weight, had battled eating disorders, relationship woes, or illness. DING, DING, DING!! That's me. I want to do this category.

The girl said it's a very laid-back category. You can wear a one piece, a two-piece, or a gorilla suit. I had Roanne make me up a sarong if I panicked the day of the show and didn't want to show my ass.

One day, when my mom and I were driving, she said, "You haven't been sick since you started this diet." She was correct. I changed my Remicade to every five weeks and was taking pain medication four times daily. Between the two changes plus my diet, I could train, be a mom, cook, clean, and rest. I had to nap every day at 1:00. I went to bed every night at 8:20. If I had the urge to eat, I would go to bed. By the end of the day, I was exhausted. Because of the water intake, I would get up, at least, six

95

times every night. During the day, I would tinkle every 30 minutes. As the show neared, the 5 a.m. workouts were getting harder, and I was getting tired. My show was the first week of November, so I still had three weeks to train and diet.

Remicade day came around, and I was sick as a dog. I spiked a fever, and the nurse debated about giving me treatment. I begged them for it. They called the doctor, and we were good to go. I thought I would die during that treatment. I felt so sick. Something seemed off with my body. I rested the next day and trained at night. I was weak. But I still trained. I was spending a lot of time in the bathroom again, spiking fevers at night. But those are common symptoms for Crohn's.

I went for my last fitting. I borrowed my cousin's prom gown, and I tried on my suit. My mom asked me if I cheated on the diet. I almost killed the old woman. The seamstress looked at my mom and said, "You never say those words to a fitness competitor."

I practiced, regularly, walking in my heels. They were five inches high. I did the dishes in them, walked the dog, and cooked and cleaned.

A week before the show, Kevin sat down and explained the entire process. It's called "peak week." My last leg workout was on a Tuesday before the show. On my first set of squats, I went to squat and felt a tearing in my hiney. I was in the gym, so I couldn't scream. I picked up all my shit and went straight home. I was bleeding because I split my rectum open. It hurt to sit down. But I had nitro cream in the house and would have eaten it if I had to.

Nitroglycerin cream is a miracle for fissures, but it causes a massive headache when you first apply it because it lowers your blood pressure. I called Kevin and told him what happened.

The day before the show, I needed spray tanning at the host hotel. I took my mom with me. When I walked in, all I could see was one stunning girl after another. Everybody was beautiful. Where the hell did they come from?

My mom was in awe. Competitors flew in from all over the United States, others flew in from out of the country.

When I got tanned, all my clothes had to come off. I never felt so naked in my life. I had to open my legs, close them, bend over, turn to the left, the back, and the side. Every inch was sprayed tanned. When I came out, my mom had struck up a conversation with a bunch of girls. They were commenting on how cute she was, how she didn't look 81.

The tan felt sticky and smelled awful. When I came home, I crawled into bed, feeling disgusting from being spray tanned. And then I prayed. I had seven hours before I had to be at the venue.

I had finished "peak weak" and was hoping I did it correctly. You dehydrate your body of all the water your body was holding onto.

When I got on the scale that morning, it read 115 pounds. I started at 152. I did it. I never worked so hard in my life at doing something outside of court reporting school.

Because I live in Rhode Island, it takes 15 minutes to get everywhere.

I arrived at the venue by 5 a.m. and had my hair and makeup done around 8:00 a.m.

After my hair and makeup were done, the inevitable was about to happen. I had to put the bikini on. I put it on, with caution, fearing I would break it. Once it was on, I had my beautiful sarong on, covering all my bits and pieces.

Suddenly, I stopped and looked around. Tits and asses surrounded me for miles. I said to myself, "You know, what, Claudia? Fuck it." I took off that sarong, put my five-inch heels on, and I walked around and mingled with the other girls.

The girls couldn't be more helpful. There were so many misconceptions about fitness competitors. They were all untrue.

I absorbed what was going on around me. Here I was, Claudia Merandi, who never wore a bathing suit in my life, I was walking around in a bikini and heels.

I always took showers in the dark because I didn't like my body. I hated to see the incisions on my stomach, and I was never comfortable being naked. If I could take a shower clothed, I would have.

But after one hour, in my bikini and heels, everybody started to look alike. I kept smacking the girls on their asses because I had never seen asses like that, except on the Kardashians.

But I, honestly, couldn't tell one girl from the next.

My category was called. We were lined up, waiting, and we all talked to one another. One girl lost 300 pounds, one girl was in an abusive relationship. The girls and the guys all had a story. Everybody's got a story. They achieved obstacles in life just like I had.

I was sitting down backstage because I had rectal pain and I was talking with one of the engineers.

I said, "Do you realize I'm talking to you half naked in heels?" He said I was a nut.

The MC had a voice like velvet. It was my time to walk. I could hear the MC reading my biography. He was so good at his job. When he said, "This is Claudia Merandi" I almost shit my pants. But something came over me. I walked out, struck a pose, and then walked into the center.

I could hear people screaming my name. The MC was still reading my bio, and I stopped posing. I looked around, and I took in every minute. I waved at people while I was on stage. Fuck the stupid posing. I was there to bring awareness to the Crohn's Colitis Community. I was blowing kisses, waving, doing everything you should never do, on stage, when you're in a fitness show. I had put in my bio that the show was dedicated to my aunt, my mom's twin, and I broke down. When he was done, I made the sign of the cross, looked up at God, and made my way backstage.

One girl said, "Girl, you just won." Won? You win something? Huh? Next, we had to put our gowns on. We came back onstage. I was so involved with everything going on, I didn't know there were winners in this category. The other girls looked so much better than me, so I automatically assumed they won.

I was smiling and waving at people, this time in my gown, and then the MC called my name. I placed in the top five, which was great.

But I already won. I was a winner. I kept saying, "I did it. I did it. I did it. I did it."

I walked backstage, got out of my gown, and said my goodbyes. I made so many wonderful friends I still talk to today.

When I made my way out to the foyer, people kept stopping me. I was looking for my kids and my mom. People kept congratulating me, telling me their stories about Crohn's, thanking me. Thanking me? Why were they thanking me?

I found my family. Everybody was screaming, hugging. It was magical. Everybody embraced me, and I enjoyed every minute of that day and night.

Once we were in the car, I was ready to eat my egg roll. The only fucking Japanese restaurant we chose didn't have egg rolls. I was too high on adrenaline to eat.

When I got home, I took off all the makeup, eyelashes, took a shower and put on my favorite white cotton nightgown.

I felt like I did the night I made my First Communion. I was too excited to sleep. But I felt different. I felt as though the next chapter in my life would differ from the past twenty-five years of my life.

THE "AFTER SHOW EXPERIENCE"

The next morning, I looked at my phone and thought I was seeing things. *Four hundred* people commented on my fitness competition. As the day went on, the numbers grew.

My mom said, "Look what you've been through. This is just another part of you." She said, "You have to get involved in a support group." She had been saying that for years, but I just blew her off. My mother is never wrong.

A few days after the show, when I woke up, I didn't feel well. I felt like my body crashed. The diarrhea was back with a vengeance. I never got my cheat meal because my stomach was bothering me. I waited another day, but I was getting worse.

I got admitted the Wednesday after the show. I was in pain, I was tired, and I felt like I had the flu. Amazingly, I had a semi-reasonable hospitalist who didn't make me beg for IV pain medication.

It was only a three-day stay, and I was treated with compassion. So, nobody would lose their medical license that week.

My body gave out. I was eating minimal amounts of food for three months, training like a beast, daily, and Crohn's came a knocking.

But over the days, I would get stronger and healthier. I knew one thing; I had a great body, and I would not revert to my old eating habits. A trainer told me, "Don't get depressed when you start packing on the weight." Not me. I wasn't packing on anything. I killed myself to get this body, and I would not lose it. My diet became a lifestyle. A lifestyle that changed my life.

Many people with Crohn's are offended when you tell them to change their diet and I was one of those people. I used to everything. But when you have Crohn's, you really need to eat clean. I don't consider how I eat and live to be a diet, I consider it to be a lifestyle.

THE C WORD...MY BLOG

I took my mom's advice, and I joined every support group I could find. Their stories were so like mine. But something was missing in every support group: humor. I met with this author, Joe Broadmeadow, and told him I wanted to write a book. He said that I should blog. I'm computer illiterate, so it seemed like it would be impossible. My sister, Maria, is a genius. Before I knew it, "The C Word" was up and running. I blogged about every aspect of Crohn's. I started from when I was a kid with Crohn's to an adult with Crohn's.

I would post my blogs on every support group. My blog is R rated, and it's loaded with fucks and sucks. When I started to write, I asked myself what kind of a writer do I want to be? I wanted to be a truthful writer. I went to college to become a court reporter, so I didn't even know if I was writing correctly. But it was a blog. Who gives a shit?

When I blogged, I would go deep. Over a twelve-month period, I had hundreds that would follow me, message me, tell me about their awful ER experiences. I would post videos, never thinking people would watch them. People from Maine to the UK and Australia would comment and many would be seeking help with the same issues I had experienced.

Before I knew it, I was advocating for people that couldn't advocate for themselves. I would be their voice. I would wake up to, sometimes, fifty messages and I would respond to every single person. I didn't care how long it took, they would hear from me.

People found humor in my blog. That was my only goal; to make people laugh. People with Crohn's suffer horribly from depression, and that's never addressed. Nobody tells you the other things that happen to you when you suffer from Crohn's Disease. Many don't know about the other aspects of Crohn's Disease. My blog was the place to discuss everything related to Crohn's. I blogged about depression, sex, fissures, kidney stones, raising kids with Crohn's, dealing with custody battles, getting disability, losing my business, and losing friends and family.

By October of 2017, I was responding to, at least, sixty people a day.

In April, I decided I would do the same fitness competition I did in 2016, but this time I would raise money for a Crohn's-related organization.

I chose Cure for IBD as the organization. I liked Chris, the founder, and 100 percent of what I raised went to research.

I had kept my weight since my first competition, so I just upped my training game. I worked harder every time I went to the gym. I represented the Crohn's community and I wanted to make them proud. There were days where I felt too sick to train, but I still made it there. I needed help on days I trained legs. I was a year older, and legs presented a challenge. My trainer, Josh, knew I was sick, so working with him put me in a safe zone. The diet that Kevin created for me became a lifestyle, not a diet.

As I write this last chapter, I just competed in my second fitness competition and I'm proud to say I raised $2200 for Cure for IBD. I cannot extend enough gratitude to all those who donated and for all your beautiful words of inspiration.

"THE BEGINNING AND THE END"

So, folks, there you have it; my story about living with Crohn's Disease and the many battles associated with it. Pooping my pants is sometimes the least of my worries when it comes to Crohn's Disease.

I needed the world to hear this story. It's not only my story, it's the story of millions who suffer from Crohn's/UC.

I pray that the opiate epidemic doesn't rob the chronic illness community of the care they deserve and receive pain relief without begging and proving that they're not a drug-seeking community.

I pray that the ER doctors and the hospitalists are educated on how to treat people with chronic illnesses and show compassion to all.

I pray that each ER doctor takes the time to review each patient's chart before the assumptions and judgments are made. I pray that "THE ER COMPASSION BILL FOR THE CHRONIC ILLNESS COMMUNITY" will get passed and the lawmakers will hear our cries for help.

I pray that all of you who suffer from this relentless illness find the strength to fight for what you believe in, to fight for your life, and to fight for the strength to survive.

Remember...you have a friend in Providence, Rhode Island.

ABOUT THE AUTHOR

Claudia Merandi is 49 years old, single, and lives in East Providence, Rhode Island with her two girls, Francesca 16, and Ava, 12. She has a brother, Billy, and a sister, Maria. Her mom, Dotty, 82, is her next-door neighbor and her closest friend.

Claudia's blog, claudiaandcrohnsdisease.wordpress.com is written weekly. Claudia is an advocate for the chronic illness community and speaks with people, daily, who suffer from Crohn's Disease and ulcerative colitis. She continues to work on getting her bill passed in the State of Rhode Island.

At the time of print, Claudia's Crohn's was in remission, but she still battles the illness. She's thankful for pain management and receives Remicade every five weeks. She looks forward to competing in 2018 in a different division; ironically, the bikini division.

Claudia's next book, a children's book, **Dotty on the Potty**, is about a little girl who suffers from Crohn's Disease.

Claudia's books are available on Amazon. She welcomes all to review and comment on her material. Please take a moment to review the book at www.amazon.com/**XXXXXXXXXXX**

Made in the USA
Middletown, DE
31 January 2019